A Practical Guide to Laryngeal Framework Surgery

A Practical Guide to Laryngeal Framework Surgery

Edited by Sharat Mohan, Kate Young, and Owen Judd

compton
PUBLISHING

Compton Publishing

This edition first published 2017 © 2017 by Compton Publishing Ltd.

Registered office: Compton Publishing Ltd, 30 St. Giles', Oxford, OX1 3LE, UK Registered company number: 07831037

Editorial offices: 35 East Street, Braunton, EX33 2EA UK Web: www.comptonpublishing.co.uk

ISBN 978-1-909082-07-6

A catalogue record for this book is available from the British Library.

Cover design: David Siddall, http://www.davidsiddall.com

Set in Adobe Caslon Pro/Myriad 12pt by Stuart Brown

1 2017

Table of Contents

Dedicated to our children:

Megha, Max, Toby, Sophie

Acknowledgements

We would like to thank all the contributing authors enabling us to produce this book. In addition, we would also like to thank the following people, without whose help the preparation of the manuscript would not have been possible:

Raguwinder Sahota
Netsebrak Zewde
Pradnya Mone-Pandit
Ross Hancock
Sara Colledge
Mark Johnston

and Keith Jones for encouraging the original concept.

List of contributors

Editors

Sharat Mohan, MB BS, MS, DLO (India), DLORCS (London), Specialist Laryngologist (retired), Royal Derby Hospital UK; Past Director British Voice Association, UK

Owen Judd, BMedSci(Hons) MB BS MRCP(Glas) FRCS(Ed) FRCS(ORL-NHS) FRSA PGDipClinEd DCH, Honorary Assistant Professor, University of Nottingham; Consultant Neurotologist and Laryngologist, Ear, Nose and Throat Surgeon, Royal Derby Hospital, UK

Kate Young, B. App Sci (Speech Pathology) Hons, FRCSLT, Clinical Lead Speech & Language Therapist Voice / Head & Neck, Derby Voice Clinic, Royal Derby Hospital UK; Past President and Treasurer, British Voice Association

Contributing authors

Theo Athanathiadis, MB BS, PhD, FRACS, Voice Specialist, Consultant ENT Surgeon, Adelaide, Australia

Smita Bangad, ENT Specialist Surgeon, Royal Derby Hospital, UK

Simon Carney, MD, FRACS, FRCS, FRCSE, Professor of Otorhinolaryngology and Consultant Surgeon, Flinders University, Australia

Declan Costello, FRCS, Consultant Laryngologist, Queen Elizabeth Hospital, Birmingham, UK

Meredydd Harries, FRCS, Consultant Laryngologist, Brighton NHS Trust, UK

Markus Hess, MD, Professor and Director, Deutsche Stimmklinik, Department of Voice, Speech and Hearing Disorders, University Medical Center of Hamburg-Eppendorf, Germany

Julian McGlashan, FRCS, Consultant ENT Surgeon and Honorary Assistant Professor, University of Nottingham, Queens Medical Centre, Nottingham, UK

Deepak Mehta, MD, Associate Professor of Otolaryngology, University of Pittsburgh School of Medicine & Children's Hospital of Pittsburgh, USA

Jayakumar Menon, DLO, DNB, MS, FRCS (Glasgow), Consultant Laryngologist, Kerala Institute of Medical Sciences (KIMS), Past President, Association of Phonosurgeons of India

Navneet Narula, Consultant Anaesthetist, Royal Derby Hospital UK

Nupur Kapoor Nerurkar, MB BS, DORL, MS(ENT), Consultant Laryngologist and Voice Surgeon, Bombay Hospital and Medical Research Center, Mumbai, India; Past President, Association of Phonosurgeons of India

Alexander Philip, Anaesthetic Registrar, Royal Derby Hospital, UK

Vyas M.N. Prasad, MD, Consultant Otolaryngologist, Head and Neck Surgeon, Alexandra Hospital, and Ng Teng Fong Hospital, Singapore

Marc Remacle, MD, PhD, Professor of Laryngology, University Hospital and Director, Voice and Swallowing Center, CHL Luxembourg

Jane Shaw, FRCSLT, Consultant Speech and Language Therapist, Doncaster Royal Infirmary, UK

James P. Thomas, MD, Consultant Laryngologist, Portland, OR, USA

Prasad John Thottam, MD, Department of Pediatric Otolaryngology-Head & Neck Surgery, Children's Hospital of Pittsburgh of UPMC, USA

Mark Watson, FRCS, Consultant ENT Surgeon, Doncaster Royal Infirmary, UK

Foreword

Laryngeal framework surgery has been at the centre of surgical management for the immobile and/or paralysed vocal fold since its development by Professor Isshiki in the 1970s. However, in recent years in the UK there has been a subtle shift in the management paradigm for vocal fold immobility from early speech therapy followed by a 'wait and see' approach, with framework surgery as the fallback, to early surgical intervention with injectable materials.

A corollary to this resurgence of interest in laryngeal injection has been a proliferation of courses designed to improve surgical competency in laryngeal injection approaches. One could easily foresee a day in the not-too-distant future in which facility and comfort with procedures utilizing injection techniques could relegate laryngeal framework procedures to the back cupboards of the armamentarium of the modern laryngologist and off the curriculum of the laryngological trainee.

This would be a substantial error. Laryngeal framework surgery has a proven evidence base for improvement in our patients' voice outcomes. Facility with framework surgery has led to a fundamental increase in our understanding of laryngeal structure and function. It is my opinion that such facility needs to remain at the very heart of laryngological education and training.

So, for the practising laryngologist, what approach to use, when to use it, and how? This practical guide, I am pleased to state, addresses these queries. It offers a detailed guide to just about every aspect of laryngeal framework surgery that the contemporary laryngologist could have whilst also supplying useful information on injection techniques. There are chapters on such areas as medialization thyroplasty, arytenoid adduction, cricothyroid approximation, laryngeal resizing for voice feminization, relaxation thyroplasty, lateralization procedures, and, yes, a chapter on injection laryngoplasty. There are chapters on history and on the future, chapters on clinical assessment, speech therapy, and anaesthesia.

It is my expectation that the reader will find him or herself reaching for this practical guide on a regular basis. I wish each of you an enjoyable read, and hope that this little gem of a book proves invaluable to your surgical practice.

John Rubin, MD, FRCS, FACS

Foreword

Exactly 100 ago in 1915, Payr published an article on a technique for medialization laryngoplasty that he had performed. The operation demonstrated that a small procedure can produce a substantial improvement in voice. During that same period (1911), Brünings published his approach to augment an immobile vocal fold in a patient with unilateral vocal fold paralysis. So, after 100 years and after a surge of phonosurgical articles and textbooks over the last 30 years, why come up with a new textbook and guide for laryngeal framework surgery and phonosurgery?

Well, even though volumes have been written about techniques for vocal improvement, specialists in our field still have the impression that these techniques are not used as frequently as they might be. Perhaps one answer lies in the assumption that phonosurgery is too complicated, or phonosurgical learning curves might be too steep and younger colleagues become demotivated or even frightened. If so, there should no longer be any excuses for not performing phonosurgical procedures. It is to the credit of the authors of this practical guide that they have sought to eradicate these inhibitions and restraints by showing us that phonosurgery in a clinical setting, with all of the prerequisites from diagnosis, anesthesia, post-operative follow-up, can be managed and how this may best be achieved.

Usefulness and practicality, together with detailed recommendations, is what beginners require. The editors have succeeded in presenting a book that is comprehensive enough to offer much practical information to the interested reader, while keeping the format of the guide portable. The task-specific chapters on techniques are really well laid out – they are short, to the point, and include tips and tricks. The chapters are very well illustrated with many figures, and the references offer a quick link to more detailed literature for the interested reader. The authors have done their best to share from their own experience, and have not excluded addressing potential risks, or avoiding mention of possible complications – and how best to deal with them.

This is an excellent piece of work for motivated colleagues who are willing to go the extra mile into this exciting and expanding field of phonosurgery.

Markus Hess, MD

Preface

On the evening of my retirement party, a colleague of mine pulled me to one side and whispered to me, "Sharat, you must write a book on voice surgery. You and Kate together have years of experience in this field. It should not be wasted."

I said, "We have already done some work on this; thanks for the idea."

I came home and gave it some serious thought. I thought, I will write up whatever work I have done with Kate. I discussed this with my fellow editors, Kate and Owen, and they were both positive. We started contacting people and at some point in time, this guide 'evolved'!

The response from potential contributors was excellent. The icing on the cake was when Kate called and said she had spoken to Markus Hess, whom we had met in London a few years before, and he not only agreed to write a Foreword to the book, but also expressed an interest in contributing a chapter. In addition to Dr Hess, we are all extremely thankful to John Rubin who wrote the other Foreword for us, and was always very supportive of our work.

Our book begins with an introduction and European Classification by Declan Costello and Owen Judd. It highlights the fact of how vital voice is in all age groups – children, professionals, and the retired – and stresses its economic impact on society. It also covers relevant history, including early publications, laryngoscopic techniques, laryngeal diseases, and treatments for vocal fold weaknesses.

The next chapter, also by Owen and Declan, details the anatomy and physiology of the larynx, featuring diagrams of the gross anatomy and histology of the vocal fold and the physiology of the mucosal wave. There is an extremely good table on the intrinsic muscles of the larynx and their actions, which was always difficult for me personally to learn as a medical student in the 1970s!

Following this, Julian McGlashan, nicely complements the previous chapter in his discussion on objective assessment and the principles of stroboscopy. He explains methods of examination and equipment in the voice clinic, the importance of digital recordings, techniques and protocols of examinations. The chapter also covers high speed digital imaging and diagnostic microlaryngoscopies. Julian also explains special situations, such as assessment of children and singers. This is a very informative chapter for doctors and speech therapists in setting up a joint voice clinic.

After this, Kate Young and Jane Shaw explain the role of speech therapists in laryngeal framework surgery. In our practice, the speech therapist has a major role and we started a trend in the UK that the speech therapist is physically present in the operating theatre for a medialization thyroplasty, as an un-scrubbed available clinician. This is very important for 'voice trials', when the surgeon places the implant under local anaesthesia. I personally have never operated on a patient without consulting and involving my speech therapist.

This chapter also explains the importance of observing the patient on the day of the procedure (in cases of injection laryngoplasty as an outpatient procedure), management of suboptimal outcomes, and long term follow-up. This is a must read chapter for surgeons and speech therapists alike.

Though the majority of laryngeal framework surgery is performed using local anaesthesia, we always had an anaesthetist in the operating theatre. The chapter on anaesthesia by Navneet Narula and A. Philip explains the importance of being aware of the initial pathology that has prompted the need for laryngeal framework surgery. It also emphasizes the residual effects causing altered laryngeal and pharyngeal anatomy, sensation, and potential effects of chemotherapy or radiotherapy. The chapter also explains issues relating to smokers, highlights the importance of suppression of airway reflexes, the cooperation of the sedated patient, awake enough to phonate on command, and, most importantly, how to approach sharing the airway with the surgeon.

It explains local anaesthesia with target controlled sedation, general anaesthesia (GA) techniques with microlaryngeal tubes (MLT) and laryngeal masks (LMA). It also stresses the importance of theatre staff being aware of the immediate post-operative problems. I thank Navneet for this excellent chapter and being part of our team.

In our chapter on type I thyroplasty, we demonstrate step-by-step, and with photographs, the way we have successfully operated in Derby for several years using custom made silicone implants. With type I medialization being the most commonly performed laryngeal framework surgery procedure across the world, I feel that it is the 'bread and butter' for the specialist framework voice surgeon; rather like tonsillectomy for a general ENT surgeon. This chapter is full of clear photographs of the procedure itself and of the common pitfalls. I thank Smita

Bangad, a good friend and colleague, for her input in this chapter and her help in the later years of my clinical career.

Marc Remacle and V. M. N. Prasad's chapter on type I medialization using the Montgomery Implant illustrates this technique in detail with brilliant text and photographs. Typically of Marc, it is very informative and explains his practice of measuring the 'Direct Peak Subglottic Pressure' (DPSGP) intra-operatively using a trans-cricothyroid catheter, which indicates the lowest subglottic pressure necessary for voicing, e.g. the lower the DPSGP, the better the voice. They also illustrate the GA technique, mentioning their preference of LMA to size 6 ET tube and the assessment of glottis closure checked with a flexi scope passed through a port in the connecting tube of the LMA.

Reflecting the wealth of experience and communication skills of the authors, Nupur Kapoor Nerurkar and Jayakumar Menon, the chapter on arytenoid adduction describes a technically challenging operation in a comprehensive way, yet which can be easily understood by beginners in voice surgery. The authors are good friends of ours and always supported our work in India.

We are extremely thankful to Mark Watson and Jane Shaw for their chapter on injection laryngoplasty. Although, strictly speaking, it is not a framework surgery, our book would have been incomplete without this contribution.

Simon Carney and Theodore Athanasiadis's chapter on type II thyroplasty very nicely describes cordectomy (Dennis & Kashima), cordotomy, and other lateralization procedures. Simon mentions the importance of enlarging the airway, while trying to avoid a major impact on vocal function. The authors review various surgical options, including cordectomy/cordotomy, arytenoidectomy, arytenoid abduction, suture lateralization, re-innervation, laryngeal pacing, and Botox injection. Simon wonders why the term 'foldotomy' is not used instead of cordotomy and we often wondered the same! I like Simon's optimism in relation to re-innervation techniques and I hope it comes true. We thank Simon, a former Derby trainee, for contributing this chapter in spite of his busy schedule in Australia.

Marc Remacle and V.M.N. Prasad describe type III thyroplasty – relaxing with a midline wedge. This procedure lowers the vocal pitch and is mainly performed for female to male transsexual patients and mutational falsetto (puberphonia) in males who do not respond to voice, or psychotherapy.

Chapters on cricothyroid approximation by Meredydd Harris and Declan Costello and laryngeal resizing by James P. Thomas describe feminization of voice by two different techniques. Cricothyroid approximation (CTA) describes transgender voice feminization and its occasional indication for androphonia. This chapter stresses the importance undertaking speech therapy for transgender patients in a specialized centre.

Laryngeal resizing by James P. Thomas illustrates this complex technique with excellent photographs, as we have come to expect from a laryngologist whom, I recall, gave a presentation on 'How to get good images of the larynx' in one of our British Voice Association educational meetings.

Vocal fold augmentation in children by Deepak Mehta and Prasad Thottam describes the paediatric larynx, which is still growing, and the differences in anatomy from the adult larynx. Based on their experience in the USA, they are of the opinion that temporary injection medialization is preferred to framework surgery. Specifically, their chapter tells you when ***not*** to undertake LFS in children. We thank Deepak, a former Derby trainee, for this chapter.

This guide ends with a chapter from Markus Hess on future techniques in phonosurgery, featuring numerous informative photographs and new ideas which are self-explanatory.

Aside from those who have contributed directly, I have to thank Professor Hans Mahieu for teaching me almost everything I learnt, allowing me to attend his clinics and operating theatre sessions at the Vrije Universiteit (VU) in Amsterdam and, more importantly, giving me the opportunity to meet and learn from the Master and the undisputed 'Father of Laryngeal Framework Surgery', Professor Nobuhiko Isshiki, during his laryngeal framework surgery courses in Amsterdam.

Special thanks go to Ragwinder (Bindy) Sahota, an ENT Speciality trainee at the Royal Derby Hospital, whose IT skills have been put to best use in tirelessly managing all images for this book.

Finally, I must thank my good friends and co-editors, Kate Young and Owen Judd, for doing all the important work during all those weekends, in spite of their busy clinical schedules and family commitments.

Sharat Mohan

SECTION I: OVERVIEW

1

Introduction and classifications

Declan Costello and Owen Judd

Introduction

A voice is vital for communication in order to work, attend education, socialize, and function at home. Voice disorders (hoarseness, voice loss or discomfort when speaking) are common in a world where 90% of all professions require a degree of voice use. In the Western world, approximately 1 in 25 (or around 40 million) of the general population will suffer from voice difficulties at some stage of their lives. In the USA alone, the National Institute on Deafness and Other Communication Disorders (NIDCD) collated statistics and reported in 2015 that an estimated 17.9 million US adults aged 18 or older, or 7.6% of the population, reported having had a problem with their voice in the past 12 months.

Of the estimated 40 million humans with voice problems in the West, statistically, 20% of children have a voice problem during their early years and one out of every five teachers in the front line of voice use will suffer from poor vocal health. After teachers, the US National Center for Voice and Speech (NCVS) reports that entertainers (singers and actors), factory workers or machine operators, managers, clerical workers, and sales personnel feature highly on their list of client referrals.

Add to this the rate of growth of the aging population, which is increasing year on year. Older people without an adequate voice risk losing their ability to work successfully as retirement ages increase and, later, face social isolation as they become less mobile and rely on telecommunications to keep in touch. In all walks of life, whether social or commercial, maintaining vocal strength during the aging process becomes further necessary in order to compensate for impaired hearing, which often also affects this population.

Disruption to vocal communication has a greater economic impact than might be expected, reflected in lost time from work and poor performance among professional voice users. The estimated cost of voice disorders to the British economy alone is approximately £200 m a year. The potential loss of work and social support produces stress and depression, which will invariably impact on general health, with further implications for individuals, care providers, companies, and national economies. These factors, among many others, have led to the clinical development and importance of voice disorders and phonosurgery worldwide over the last few centuries.

History

The first known published essay on diseases of the larynx was written by Giovanni Codronchi of Italy in 1597. However, it wasn't until three years later that a full account of the larynx as a vocal organ, *De Larynge vocis organo*, was published by Hieronymus ab Aquapendente. The first laryngoscope, or 'glottiscope', was presented to the Hunterian Society in London by Benjamin Guy Babbington in 1829. In 1855, an adaptation of this device, utilizing reflected sunlight, was presented to the Royal Society of London in a paper entitled 'Observations on the Human Voice' by Manuel Garcia. This technique sparked a great interest in the new specialty of laryngology and Garcia became regarded as the 'father' of the field. He went on to have honours bestowed upon him by other great physicians of the time, including a great celebration of his 100th birthday in 1905, which was attended by laryngologists from all over the world.

In 1859, Sir Morell MacKenzie began to master laryngoscopic techniques and established a rapidly developing laryngology practice. In 1863, he won the Jackson Prize of the Royal College of Surgeons of England with his paper, 'The Pathology and Treatment of Laryngeal Disease', and went on to publish the first great textbook of laryngology in 1865: *The Use of the Laryngoscope in Diseases of the Throat*. He was just 26 years of age and had established a reputation as the leading laryngologist in the UK. He is still regarded as one of the great pioneers in ear, nose, and throat surgery.

Vocal fold paralysis was first studied formally in Berlin in 1863, by Carl Gerhardt. He discovered that the majority of such cases were due to recurrent laryngeal nerve lesions. The mechanism of paralysis and the vocal fold positions were later described by German physician, Ottomar Rosenbach, in 1880. His name was attributed to the Semon–Rosenbach Law, often referred to as simply 'Semon's Law', that the abductor fibres of the recurrent laryngeal nerve are affected first in palsy, with the adductor fibres being initially spared.

Surgical treatment to restore the function of a paralysed vocal fold was not initially thought possible; however, in 1939, the first successful operative procedure was performed by Brian King in Seattle, USA. He proceeded to publish his work on the subject. Subsequently, various techniques for safe surgery on the skeleton, or framework, of the larynx were developed.

Originally described by Payr in 1915, the term 'laryngeal framework surgery' (LFS) refers to surgical procedures performed on the laryngeal skeleton, comprising the thyroid, cricoid and arytenoid cartilages, with the aim of altering the position and/or the tension of the vocal folds. From a functional point of view, LFS may serve to alter the vibratory movements of the vocal folds in such a way as to reduce glottal insufficiency (thus to reduce breathiness), or to change the pitch of voice.

However, in the pre-antibiotic era, complications were common and the concept was largely abandoned. Over the following decades, the surgical techniques were modified and evolved and, in 1974, Nobuhiko Isshiki of Kyoto University, Japan, described 'Thyroplasty as a new phonosurgical technique'. This seminal research, performed in the canine model, outlined the four types of LFS, below, that we currently recognize. Thus, Isshiki can be seen as the 'father' of modern laryngeal framework surgery. Isshiki described the importance of surgery under local anaesthesia in order to obtain constant vocal feedback from the patient. He went on to develop the now widely used Isshiki Classification for Laryngeal Framework Surgery.

Classifications

Isshiki described four basic surgical procedures that he called thyroplasty types I–IV. He also described arytenoid adduction, which aims to close the posterior glottis. The four types were

- thyroplasty type I (medialization)
- thyroplasty type II (lateralization)
- thyroplasty type III (relaxing)
- thyroplasty type IV (tensing).

In 2001, the Phonsurgery Commitee of the European Laryngological Society (ELS) produced a classification and nomenclature system that incorporated Isshiki's own descriptions from 1974, and added further procedures that had been developed in the intervening years:

- Approximation laryngoplasty
  - Medialization thyroplasty
    - (Thyroplasty type I)
  - Arytenoid adduction
    - *Rotation (pull) techniques*
      - (Lateral cricoarytenoid pull technique)
    - *Fixation techniques*
      - (Adduction arytenopexy)

- Expansion laryngoplasty
  - Lateralistion thyroplasty
    - *Lateral approach*
      - (Thyroplasty type IIa)
    - *Medial approach*
      - (Thyroplasty type IIb, expansion of the anterior commissure, midline lateralization thyroplasty)
  - Vocal fold abduction
    - Suture technique
    - Resection technique
    - (Thyroarytenoid myectomy)

- Relaxation laryngoplasty
  - Shortening thyroplasty
    - *Lateral approach*
      - (Thyroplasty type III)
    - *Medial approach*
      - (Anterior commissure retrusion)

- Tensioning laryngoplasty
  Cricothyroid approximation
    (Thyroplasty type IVa, cricothyroid subluxation)
  Elongation thyroplasty
    Lateral approach
      (Thyroplasty type IVb)
    Medial approach
      (Springboard advancement, anterior commissure advancement, anterior commissure laryngoplasty)

LFS has been applied in numerous different circumstances, with the most commonly performed procedure being a type I thyroplasty, primarily an operation for glottal insufficiency, that aims to maximize glottal closure during phonation, cough, and swallow.

Prior to discussion of the nuances of LFS, it is necessary to have a precise and detailed understanding of laryngeal anatomy and physiology as described in the next chapter.

Further reading

Babington BG. 1829. Lecture to the Hunterian Society. *London Medical Gazette* 3:555.

Friedrich G, de Jong FI, Mahieu HF, et al. 2001. Laryngeal framework surgery: a proposal for classification and nomenclature by the Phonosurgery Committee of the European Laryngological Society. *Eur Arch Otorhinolaryngol* **258**(8):389–96.

Garcia M. 1854–5. Observations on the human voice. *Proc R Soc Lond* 7:399–410.

Isshiki N, Morita H, Okamura H, Hiramoto M. 1974. Thyroplasty as a new phonosurgical technique. *Acta Otolaryngol* **78**(5–6):451–7.

Isshiki N, Tanabe M, Ohkawa M, Kita M. 1985. Laryngeal framework surgery for voice disorders. *Auris Nasus Larynx* **12** Suppl 2:S217–20.

King BT. 1939. A new and function-restoring operation for bilateral abductor cord paralysis, a preliminary report. *Tr Amer Laryngol* **61**:264–96.

MacKenzie M. 1865. *The Use of the Laryngoscope in Diseases of the Throat, with an appendix on rhinoscopy.* London: Churchill.

Sebastian, A. 1999. *A Dictionary of the History of Medicine.* New York, NY: Parthenon Publishing.

Wright J. 1914. *A History of Laryngology and Rhinology.* Philadelphia, PA: Lea & Febiger.

2

Anatomy and physiology of the larynx

Owen Judd and Declan Costello

Anatomy

The larynx is composed of three elements: the skeleton, the mucosal layer, and the muscles.

The laryngeal skeleton

The skeleton of the larynx is composed of a single bone, the hyoid, and nine cartilages. There are three unpaired cartilages: the thyroid, cricoid, and epiglottic; and three paired: the arytenoid, corniculate, and cuneiform.

The hyoid

The hyoid bone (Figure. 2.1) suspends the cartilaginous skeleton of the larynx and is itself suspended from the skull by the suprahyoid muscles. The function of the hyoid is to elevate and lower the larynx during phonation and changes in pitch. It consists of a central body and two pairs of horns, or cornu – the lesser and greater – and is connected to the thyroid cartilage by the thyrohyoid muscles, membrane, and ligaments.

The thyroid cartilage

The thyroid cartilage (Figure. 2.2) makes up the greatest part of the laryngeal skeleton. It comprises two flat plates of hyaline cartilage which meet in the midline and form the laryngeal prominence. Superiorly in the midline there is a depression, named the superior thyroid notch, and a corresponding inferior

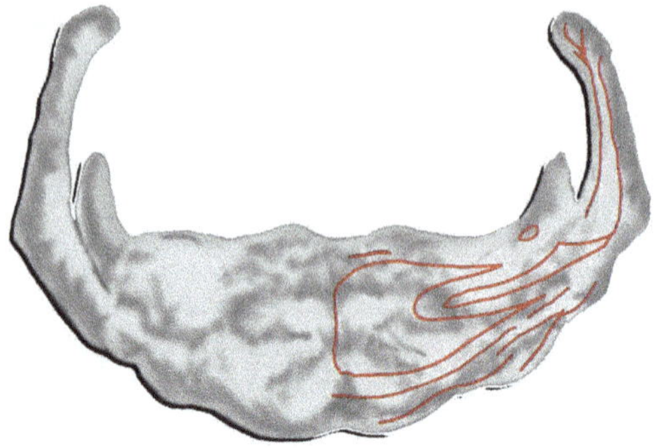

Figure. 2.1: Hyoid showing muscle attachments, seen from above. Author image.

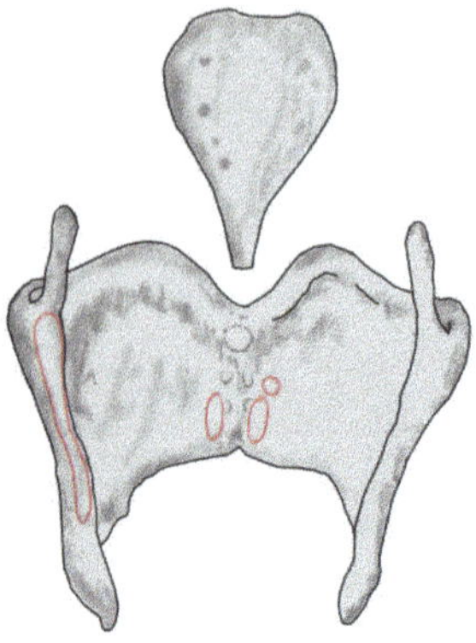

Figure. 2.2: Muscle attachments on thyroid cartilage and epiglottis, seen from the rear. Author image.

thyroid notch at its lower border. Posteriorly, there are superior and inferior thyroid horns, or cornu. The superior cornu takes attachment of the thyrohyoid ligament. The inferior cornu articulates with the cricoid cartilage, as do the posterior lower edges of the thyroid cartilage, to form the cricothyroid joints. These synovial joints move with action of the cricothyroid muscle. The whole superior border of the thyroid cartilage is suspended from the hyoid bone by the thyrohyoid membrane. The thryohyoid muscle is attached along the oblique line of the laminae.

The cricoid cartilage

This ring of hyaline cartilage is shaped as a 'signet ring' with the narrow section anteriorly placed and a broader lamina posteriorly. It is the only complete ring of cartilage in the airway. The cricoid (Figure. 2.3) is positioned immediately inferior to the thyroid cartilage and is attached to it anteriorly by the cricothyroid ligament and membrane and articulates directly with the thyroid cartilage posteriorly at the cricothyroid joint. The cricothyroid muscle originates from this cartilage anterolaterally and fans outwards and upwards to attach to the lower border and inferior

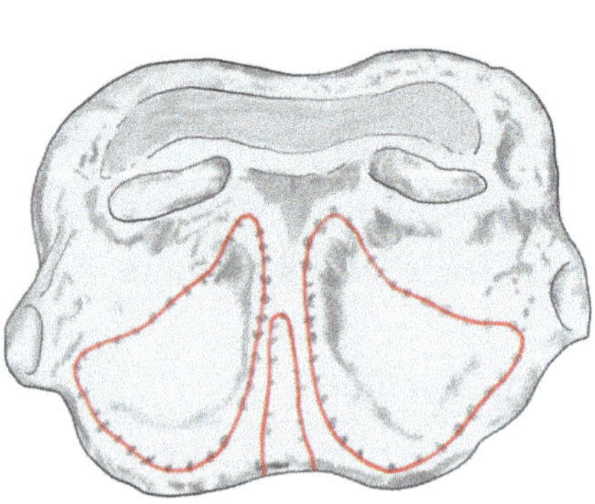

Figure. 2.3: Cricoid cartilage. Author image.

cornu of the thyroid cartilage. The cricoid cartilage is also the origin of posterior cricoarytenoid and lateral cricoarytenoid muscles. The posterior superior border of the cricoid cartilage is the articular surface for the arytenoid cartilages.

The epiglottic cartilage

This is a leaf-shaped extension of elastic cartilage attached to the internal laminae of the thyroid cartilage in the midline. During swallowing, as the hyoid elevates the larynx, the epiglottis flattens and closes over the laryngeal inlet to provide protection against aspiration.

The arytenoid cartilages

These paired cartilages (Figure 2.4) are the main functioning elements of voice production and vocal fold movement. They dictate the position and tension of the vocal folds. The arytenoids are pyramid-shaped structures of hyaline cartilage which articulate from their base as a synovial joint with the posterolateral surface of the cricoid. They have three surfaces: the posterior surface and lateral border provide origin of the oblique and transverse interarytenoid muscles which traverse the posterior larynx to attach to the other arytenoid cartilage. On the anterolateral surface of the cartilage is a ridge which curves downwards and anteriorly to form a medial process. This is termed the 'vocal process' and gives attachment to the vocal ligament, a band of yellow elastic tissue which spans the glottis and attaches into the midpoint of the posterior midline of the thyroid cartilage. The anterior surface and base of the cartilages provide attachment of the thyroarytenoid muscle. The lateral angle of the base of the cartilage points backwards and laterally to form the 'muscular process'. This is where the posterior cricoarytenoid and lateral cricoarytenoid muscles attach. The apex of the arytenoid cartilages form an articulation with the corniculate cartilages.

The corniculate and cuneiform cartilages

These small elastic paired cartilage structures form the tip of the arytenoids (Figure 2.5) and most medial aspect of the aryepiglottic folds respectively. They serve to stiffen and strengthen the mucosal folds.

Mucosa of the larynx

The majority of the mucosal surface of the larynx and pharynx above the level of the vocal folds is of stratified squamous epithelial type. Below the level of the

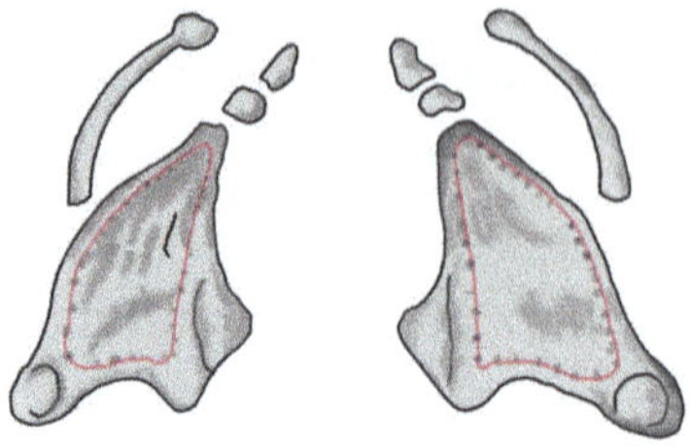

Figure 2.4: Arytenoids with corniculate and cuneiform cartilages. Author image.

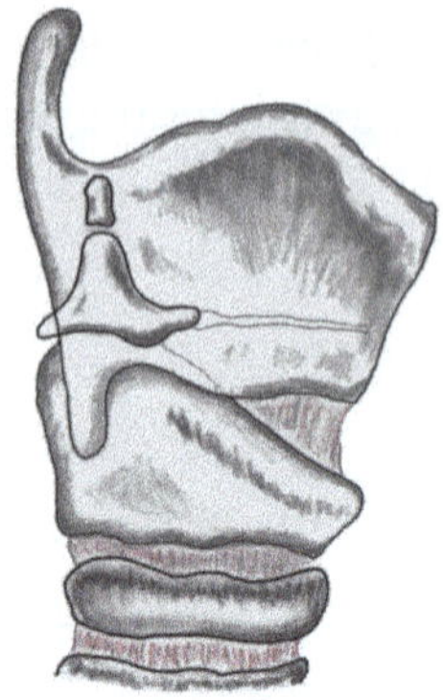

Figure 2.5: Lateral view of the laryngeal framework. Author image.

vocal folds, goblet cells are present to produce mucus and the mucosa changes to a pseudostratified ciliated columnar epithelium.

The structure of the vocal folds themselves is highly specialized and unique. They consist of five layers:

1. Epithelium – non-keratinizing stratified squamous epithelium.
2. Superficial lamina propria (Reinke's space) – loose fibrous tissue and gel matrix.
3. Intermediate lamina propria – mainly elastin fibres with some fibroblasts.
4. Deep lamina propria – mainly collagen and rich in fibroblasts.
5. Thyroarytenoid/vocalis muscle complex.

Generally speaking, the first two layers form the vibratory surface or 'cover' of the vocal fold, with the gelatinous consistency of Reinke's space allowing fluency of epithelial vibration and a free-flowing mucosal wave.

The intermediate and deep layers of the lamina propria form a transitional zone and together make up the vocal ligament. The body of the vocal fold consists mainly of the muscular layer (Figure 2.6).

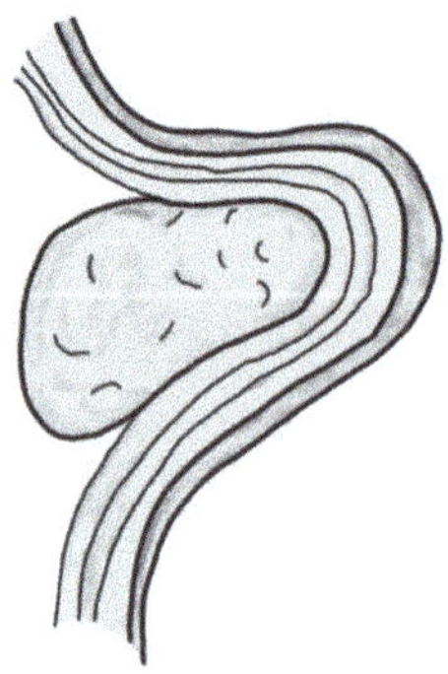

Figure 2.6: Vocal fold edge demonstrating cover, transition layer, and body of the thyroarytenoid muscle (from outwards to inwards). Author image.

The muscles

The main actions of the muscles of the larynx are: adduction (closure), abduction (opening), tensing, and shortening (Figure 2.7 and Figure 2.8).

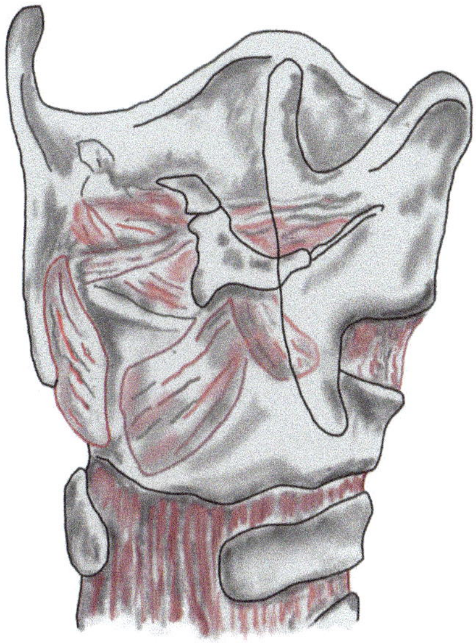

Figure 2.7: Posterolateral view of the laryngeal framework. Author image.

Adductors

Thyroarytenoid The thyroarytenoid muscle has two parts. The medial and deeper compartment is termed the vocalis muscle and lies parallel to and adherent to the vocal ligament. It forms the main part of the body of the vocal fold. The lateral compartment is termed muscularis, thyroepiglotticus or ventricularis muscle. It is attached to the edges of the epiglottis and ventricle.

Lateral cricoarytenoid This muscle is one of two which arise from the cricoid and attach into the muscular process of the arytenoid, and has an antagonistic action with the other muscle, the posterior cricoarytenoid. It is the major adductor of the vocal folds.

Interarytenoid The interarytenoid muscle comprises two separate muscle sections, the transverse and oblique arytenoid muscles. Both muscles run from one arytenoid to the other posteriorly.

Abductors

Posterior cricoarytenoid This is the only pair of muscles that abduct the vocal folds. They are also described as respiratory muscles for that reason. They are exactly antagonistic to the lateral cricoarytenoids above.

Tensors

Cricothyroid This muscle is responsible for opposing the cricoid and thyroid cartilages via backward tilt of the cricothyroid joints. The cricothyroid tenses the folds and so increases the pitch of the voice.

Thyroarytenoid Contraction of the thyroarytenoid muscle results in shortening of the vocal folds, and causes an increase in stiffness.

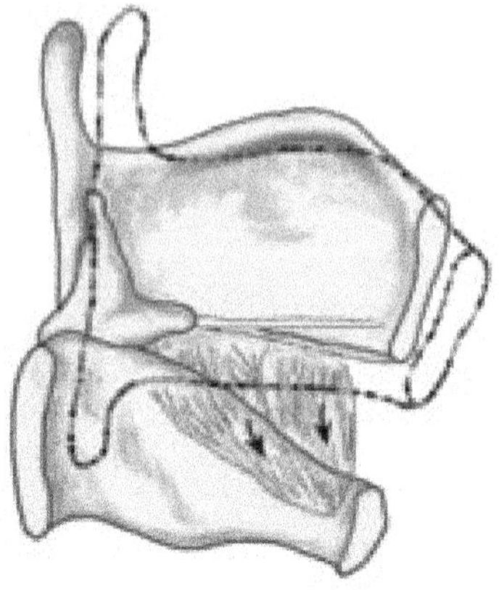

a

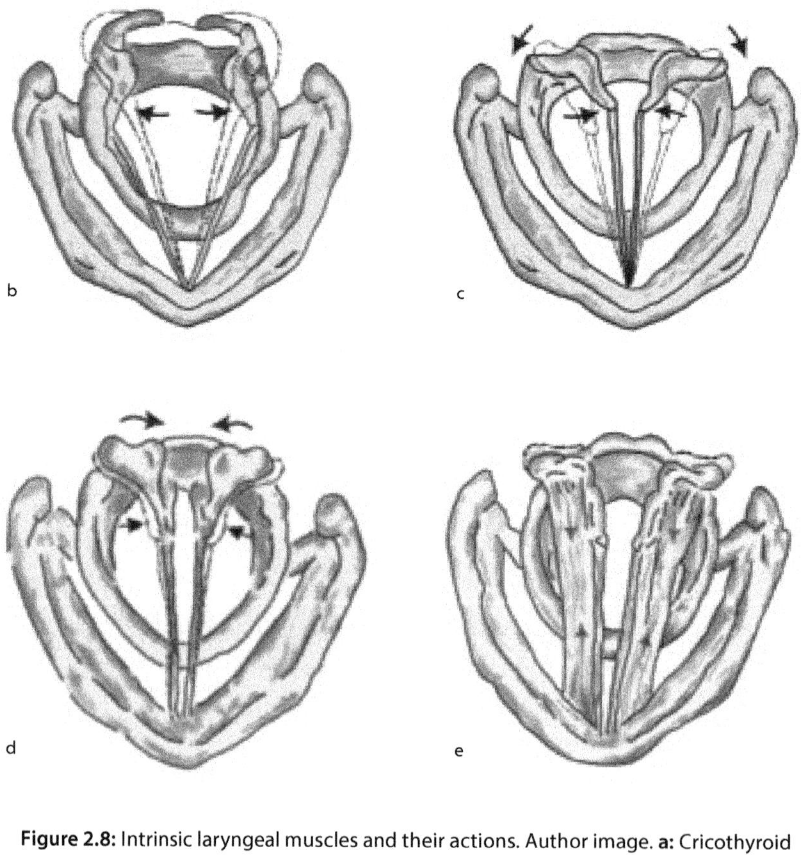

b

c

d

e

Figure 2.8: Intrinsic laryngeal muscles and their actions. Author image. **a:** Cricothyroid muscle. **b:** Posterior cricoarytenoid muscle (PCA). **c:** Lateral cricoarytenoid muscle (LCA). **d:** Interarytenoid muscle (IA). **e:** Thyroarytenoid muscle (TA).

Table 2.1: Summary of laryngeal muscles and their actions

Muscle	Origin	Insertion	Action on vocal folds	Effect on voice
Thyroarytenoid	Lower midline internal thyroid lamina	Anterior surface and base of arytenoid	Adducts, shortens, thickens, lowers, narrows laryngeal inlet Cover – slackened Body – stiffened	Enables voicing Lowers pitch Enables cough
Lateral cricoarytenoid	Lateral cricoid	Anterior surface of muscular process of arytenoid	Adducts, elongates, lowers, thins Cover – tightened Body – stiffened, edge of fold sharpened	Enables voicing Sharpens voiced sounds Whisper (when used in isolation)
Transverse interarytenoid	Lateral margin of arytenoid	Lateral margin of contra-lateral arytenoid	Adducts, medial compression of posterior glottis Cover – stabilized Body – neutral	Enables voicing Falsetto
Oblique interarytenoid	Base of arytenoid	Apex of contralateral arytenoid	Adducts, medial compression of posterior glottis, narrows laryngeal inlet Cover – neutral Body – neutral	Enables voicing Falsetto Enables cough

Muscle	Origin	Insertion	Action on vocal folds	Effect on voice
Posterior cricoarytenoid	Posterolateral face of cricoid lamina	Posterior surface of muscular process of arytenoid	Abducts, elongates, elevates, thins Cover – tightened Body – stiffened, edge of fold rounded	Disables voicing Inspiration/breathing
Cricothyroid	Anterolateral arch of cricoid	Two bellies: Oblique attaches to posterior half thyroid lamina and inferior cornu Vertical attaches to inferior border of thyroid lamina	Elongates, lowers, tenses, thins Cover – tightened Body – stiffened, edge of fold sharpened	Raises pitch

Nerve supply

The neural supply to the larynx derives from the vagus nerve, the tenth cranial nerve. The vagus gives off two main branches to the larynx, the superior laryngeal nerve (SLN), and the recurrent laryngeal nerve (RLN).

Superior laryngeal nerve

This nerve has two branches: internal and external. The internal laryngeal nerve provides sensory innervation to the mucosal surface of the larynx above the level of the vocal folds. The external laryngeal nerve supplies a single muscle – the cricothyroid. Therefore lesions of the superior laryngeal nerve present with inability to raise the pitch of the voice and coughing/choking episodes due to lack of supraglottic sensation.

Recurrent laryngeal nerve

The nerves to the left and right have different paths. The left RLN descends into the chest and hooks around the arch of the aorta to ascend back to the larynx. On the right, however, the RLN does not descend into the chest but loops around the right subclavian artery at the root of the neck. The RLN innervates all the intrinsic laryngeal muscles, except the cricothyroid, and supplies sensation from the vocal folds inferiorly. Lesions of the RLN therefore lead to vocal fold palsy.

Physiology of the laryngeal framework

Functions of the larynx

The human larynx fulfils three main functions: airway protection, respiration, and phonation. In addition, the larynx is used for coughing to expel foreign material from the airway, and for the Valsalva manoeuvre (when straining).

Protection of the airway during swallowing is achieved by closure of the true and false vocal folds, elevation of the larynx, and posterior reflection of the epiglottis to close the laryngeal inlet.

During normal quiet respiration, the vocal folds are in an abducted position, with the posterior cricoarytenoid in tonic contraction. During deep inspiration, the vocal folds abduct more widely.

Phonation and speech

The production of intelligible speech relies on a complex interaction between several different structures:

- the lungs provide an energy source;
- the vocal folds produce sound by vibrating;
- the pharynx, oral cavity and other areas modulate the resonant frequencies; and
- the mouth, soft palate and lips provide articulation.

All of these functions must be intricately coordinated for speech to be produced.

During phonation, the adductors of the vocal folds cause approximation of the arytenoid cartilages, bringing the vocal folds into close proximity. Airflow from the lungs causes vibration of the vocal folds, producing acoustic energy (sound).

The vibratory cycle of the vocal folds is described as a 'mucosal wave': pressure of air from the lungs builds under the closed vocal folds, and when the pressure exceeds the glottic closure forces, air escapes between the vocal folds. The elasticity of the vocal folds causes the vocal folds then to close again a fraction of a second later, and the vibratory cycle starts again. The closure of the vocal folds is augmented by the Bernoulli effect (in which a fluid or gas passing between two surfaces causes a negative pressure between those surfaces – in other words, the flow of air causes the side walls (the vocal folds) to tend to come together).

When viewed in coronal section (Figure 2.9), the mucosal wave is seen to propagate from inferiorly to superiorly: initially, just the most inferior margins of the vocal folds move apart. The superior borders of the vocal folds

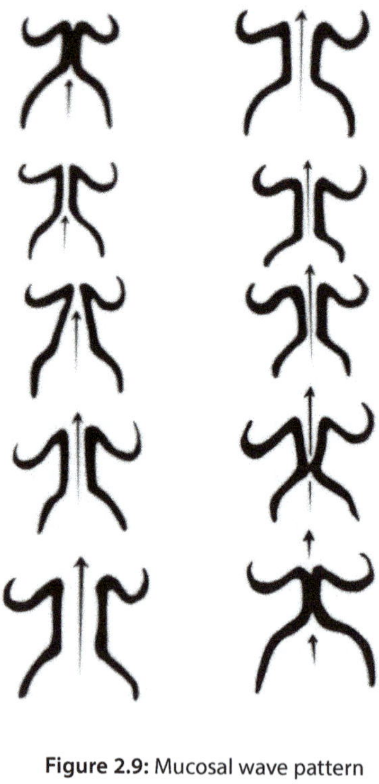

Figure 2.9: Mucosal wave pattern coronal view. Author image.

then open; the inferior surfaces then close, followed by the superior surfaces. The cycle then starts again.

The epithelial cover of the vocal folds is separated from the (relatively) stiff ligament by Reinke's space. It is this loose collagenous layer that allows the epithelium to glide over the ligament in a smooth fashion. When viewed in slow motion, this appears as a mucosal wave.

The production of a normal vocal quality relies on:

1. **Closure of the glottis.** Failure of adduction of one or both vocal folds results in poor closure and, hence, a breathy sound.
2. **Vocal folds with straight edges.** Complete closure of the glottis requires epithelial surfaces that are free from irregularities on their medial edges.
3. **A normal mucosal wave.** Any areas of the vocal fold in which there is tethering between the epithelium and the ligament will result in a non-vibratory portion of vocal fold. This results in failure vocal fold vibration that is perceived as a 'rough' quality of voice.

The pitch of voice (frequency of vibration) produced by the vocal folds is a function of:

1. **Mass per unit length.** Stretching the vocal fold results in a reduction in mass per unit length and an increase in pitch. This happens when the cricothyroid muscle contracts. Conversely, when the thyroarytenoid muscle contracts, the vocal folds shorten and increase in mass per unit length; the pitch falls.
2. **Stiffness.** Increasing the tension in the vocal fold (for example, isometric contraction, in which both thyroarytenoid and cricothyroid are working 'against' each other) alters the vibratory qualities and pitch of the vocal fold.

Different forms of laryngeal framework surgery can be employed to: increase the tension on the vocal folds, mimicking the cricothyroid muscle (as in type IV thyroplasty, cricothyroid approximation); or to medialize a paralysed vocal fold that is failing to close the glottis (as in type I thyroplasty). Equally, the vocal folds can be shortened (as in type III thyroplasty).

3

Voice therapy assessment and management

Kate Young and Jane Shaw

Introduction

The role of the Speech and Language (Voice) Therapist or Pathologist (SLT/SLP) in the voice clinic and in the wider management of surgical voice patients has modernized and developed in parallel with laryngologists' advances in patient treatment and management. The team approach to assessment, measurement, and management is essential when working with voice disordered patients.

The responsibility of the voice clinicians (both laryngologist and SLT) is to provide an accurate diagnosis and avoid inappropriate management at all stages of patient care. Cases involving those with voice disorders are often complex, with multiple factors affecting a patient's voice. Some patients will also have co-occurring swallowing difficulties.

Comprehensive assessment (physical and functional) of the disordered voice and as appropriate, swallowing, is essential before planning surgical management. Consistent assessment measures inform management planning but also enable a clinician to reflect on individual cases or whole caseloads to inform evidence-based improved clinical practice.

Voice assessment

In clinical practice, the purpose of assessment is to analyse, evaluate, and gather relevant information about the patient and the voice problem with which they present. Diagnosis and management planning is based on assessment findings and essential information regarding the impact of the voice problem. A significantly dysphonic patient may not be concerned with his or her voice quality, but a singer with a mild change in voice performance may be very anxious about their voice change and prognosis.

In addition to a full ENT examination (including palpation of the neck and a lower cranial nerve assessment where necessary), all patients should have a fibreoptic nasendoscopy and laryngoscopy. We recommend videolaryngostroboscopy (VLS) with recording facilities, using either a flexible or rigid scope, to provide a better assessment of the glottic gap, regularity of vocal fold vibration and mucosal wave.

The laryngeal examination, preferably with stroboscopy (see Chapter 4), and voice evaluation are inseparable. The laryngologist and SLT will correlate the sound of the patient's voice with visual assessment of the dysphonia presentation and must have knowledge of the extent to which the patient's abnormal voice quality is congruent with the physical findings.

A distinction needs to be made between 'data collection' and 'interpretation of findings'. Both are important, but poor assessment outcome and planning will result from omitting to complete both. It is not necessary to amass large quantities of data but, rather, to assess systematically and document essential vocal parameters and behaviours. There are assessment protocols that are useful to follow for consistency of practice.

The basic stages of voice assessment as described by Bless (1991) are:

1. interviewing;
2. observing;
3. describing the voice;
4. comparing observations to standards and normal values; and
5. integrating the information to determine treatment.

The protocol recommended by the Committee on Phoniatrics of the European Laryngological Society is a multidimensional set of minimal basic measurements suitable for all 'common' dysphonias. It consists of five different aspects:

- perception (grade, roughness, breathiness);
- videostroboscopy (closure, regularity, mucosal wave, and symmetry);
- acoustics (jitter, shimmer, F0-range, and softest intensity);
- aerodynamics (phonation quotient); and
- subjective rating (Voice Handicap Index – VHI, Visual Analogue Scale – VAS)

Case history

During this stage of evaluation, the clinician is also required to make subjective observations of the patient's voice quality, variability, the patient's emotional state, and the patient's perception of their voice problem. At the end of the assessment process, the voice clinician should understand what the patient wishes to gain from intervention and ensure that both agree to the same voice goals.

Table 3.1 desribes the data that the voice clinician should collect to complete the patient's case history, and Box 3.1 provides an example of a voice therapy assessment form.

Table 3.1: General data required from case history. From Jones, *Laryngeal Endoscopy and Voice Therapy*, Compton Publishing (2016). Courtesy of Sue M. Jones.

Feature	Detail
Personal information	Age, gender, occupation
Onset of dysphonia	Sudden
	Gradual over days/weeks/months
Progression of dysphonia	Improving/worsening over time
	Variability/consistency
	Episodic/intermittent
	Exacerbating/relieving factors
Patient's main concern	Voice quality/vocal stamina/change in range of volume/ throat pain or discomfort/fear of throat cancer/inability to sing/time off work/comments by friends or family/ unconcerned
Voice use	Home/work/social

Feature	**Detail**
Previous/ongoing medical history	Diagnosed medical conditions or undiagnosed medical symptoms: respiratory/neurological/gastrointestinal/neurological
	Upper respiratory tract infections: occasional/frequent
	Dysphagia
	Nasal symptoms
	Hearing loss
	Thyroid disorders
	Jaw/dental problems
	Allergies
	Trauma/accidents/injuries
	Surgery: laryngeal/other
	Intubation
	Menstrual cycle
Reflux symptoms	Throat clearing/throat mucus/unpleasant taste in the mouth or throat/burning throat
Current medication	Presribed and non-prescribed
Lifestyle issues	Smoking: active and passive
	Alcohol consumption
	Recreational drugs
	Environmental irritants
	Weight
Vocal care	Hydration
	Diet
	Caffeine intake
Stress and anxiety	Family dynamics
	Major life events
	Emotional

Box 3.1: Voice therapy assessment form

VOICE EVALUATION

Name:
Address:
Phone number:
Referred by:
Examiner:

Date:
Date of birth:
Age:
Occupation / student:

A. HISTORY

1. Description of the problem and cause

2. Onset and duration of the problem

3. Do you associate changes in your voice with anything in your life?

4. Variation / consistency of voice problem
   Consistancy
   Better situations
   Worse situations

5. Description of vocal use (Do you need to use your voice for your job / hobbies?)

6. Surgery (phonosurgery / general surgery) and injuries

7. Family history of speech and voice problems

8. Previous voice therapy / voice coaching / singing lessons

9. General health (including hearing, vision, allergies, asthma, etc.)

10. Swallowing / acid indigestion

B. PHYSICAL ASSESSMENT

1. Type of breathing

Clavicular	Abdominal	Thoracic
Shortness of breath	Audible breathing	Stridor

2. Breath control — On one breath:

Counts up to: ______

Sustains (number of seconds)

sss ______ zzz ______ ah ______ ee ______

3. Oral examination

Lips

Teeth

Mandibular movement

Hard and soft palate

Tongue (movement)
(diadokokinesis; ptk – ptk)

Articulation problems

4. Posture: head and neck

Face

Mandible / jaw symmetry

Neck / shoulders

General body (including posture)

5. Vocal tract discomfort: self-rating scale

Please mark the line according to the level of discomfort you are experiencing (left, right, both)

1	2	3	4	5
No discomfort	**Slight discomfort**	**Moderate discomfort**	**Severe discomfort**	**Pain**

i. Is the throat discomfort: constant intermittent variable in severity

ii. Does it occur when you are: talking at rest swallowing

iii. Tick the words that describe your throat symptoms:

burning	aching	tickling	dry
tight	irritable	sore	lump in the throat

6. Palpatory checklist

	Neutral		Hypertonic	Tenderness	
Tongue base:	1	2	3	R/L	R/L
(Geniohyoid, mylohyoid)					
Suprahyoid muscles:	1	2	3	R/L	R/L
(Digastric, etc.)					
Thyrohyoid muscles:	1	2	3	R/L	R/L
Constrictor muscles:	1	2	3	R/L	R/L
Cricothyroid muscles:	1	2	3	R/L	R/L
Strap / extrinsic muscles:	1	2	3	R/L	R/L
(SCM, omohyoid, sturnohyoid)					
Sub occipital	1	2	3	R/L	R/L

	Open	Neutral	Closed
Cricothyroid visor:	1	2	3

Laryngeal position and alignment:

Hyoid / thyroid	Aligned	Hyoid prominent	Hyoid retracted
Crico / thyroid	Aligned	Cricoid prominent	Cricoid retracted

Laryngeal movement in speech:

Neutral	Raised	Lowered	Backed
Fronted	Raised / fronted	Raised / backed	

C. CHARACTERISTICS OF VOICE

TAPE RECORDINGS – DATES:

* 0 = normal; 1 = mild; 2 = mild–moderate; 3 = moderate; 4 = moderate–severe; 5 = severe

Give score 0–5 GRBAS (Description of voice)	1st recording	2nd recording	3rd recording
G – GRADE or degree of vocal abnormality			
R – ROUGHNESS harshness heard – noise ++ mucosal wave disruption nodule/polyp/stiffness			
B – BREATHINESS tight larynx, i.e. whispery – air escape due to incomplete closure bowed VF			
A – ASTHENIC/WEAK excessive air escape VF palsy/ hypo-functional larynx			
S – STRAINED vocal fry/creak, long closed phase in vibratory cycle, hyper-adduction – arytenoid mvt +++			

1. <u>Loudness</u>

Normal ________ Too loud _______ Too soft ________ Varies _______

2. <u>Related observations</u> *

Pitch breaks ______________________ Phonation breaks ________________

Hard glottal attack _________________ Glottal fry ______________________

3. Pitch

Range: Lowest ________ Highest ________ Habitual _______

Range:

Most prominent vocal feature: ________________________

Differentiated control of seven discrete parameters of larynx and vocal tract

Larynx	Palate	Anchoring	Pharynx		
Vocal folds	Velar port	I II	Length	Tongue	Aryepiglottis
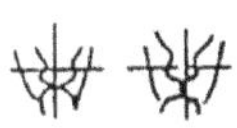	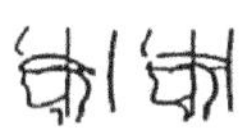	Head & Neck Torso	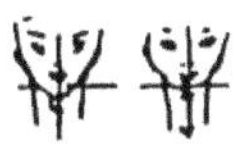	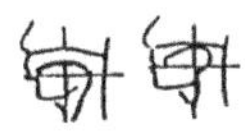	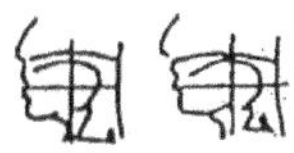
Thin – Thick	Open – Closed	Relaxed/Active	Short – Long	Relaxed – Tense	Relaxed – Narrowed
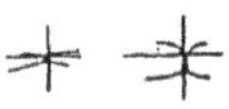	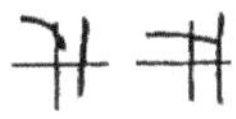	R/A R/A	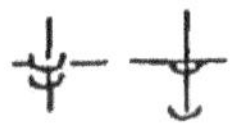	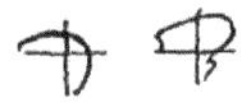	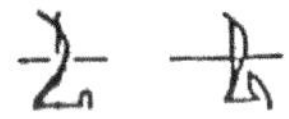

4. Clinical impressions

5. Diagnosis

6. Summary and recommendations

7. Patient specified outcome measures

Health Benefit:

Date: Goal:

Significant disruption					Optimum reached
0	1	2	3	4	5

Date: Outcome:

Significant disruption					Optimum reached
0	1	2	3	4	5

Signed ______________________________ Dated ______________________________

Patient reported impact – questionnaires (quality-of-life measures)

Self-report questionnaires enable to the clinician to understand to what extent a patient feels their voice problem is affecting their personal and/or work life. It is a useful process to determine whether a patient will engage in voice therapy and to measure voice outcome and progress in treatment.

Prior to the speech and language therapy or voice clinic appointment, patients are asked to fill out a questionnaire regarding their voice problem as they see it, detailing onset, duration, variation, recovery, and chronology of symptoms. A patient's reported voice disorder impact on their day to day activity is an essential assessment step to understand the issues fully that a patient brings to clinic and to be able to discuss what it is he or she would like the treating clinician to help with.

Quality-of-life (QOL) measures are used in specialist voice clinics and include the Voice Handicap Index (VHI)30/10, Reflux Symptom Index (RSI), Voice Symptom Scale (VoiSS), Voice-Related Quality of Life (V-RQOL), and Voice Skills Perceptual Profile (VSPP). If no sinister pathology is present, management can be guided by the perceived impact of the voice problem. A patient who scores their voice impact inappropriately high, as compared to the clinician's evaluation of their voice, may have significant psychological overlay or poor perceptual skills, both of which will need to be addressed before surgery is offered in the treatment process. Box 3.2 provides a pro forma voice clinic questionaire.

Psychoacoustic/subjective evaluation of voice

Clinicians use a variety of assessments to understand a voice problem and to plan management. Perceptual evaluation of voice is just as essential and an equally important part of the voice assessment protocol as objective voice measurement. Psychoacoustic refers to assessments that provide subjective and descriptive information about voice quality and function. The system of analysis should be consistent, repeatable, and have intra and inter rater reliability.

The vocal features being described include:

- aphonic/intermittent aphonia;
- hyperfunctional/tense;
- vocal fry/creak;
- grating;
- phonatory breaks;
- rough;
- diplophonic;
- instability of vocal pitch and/or volume; and
- pitch (appropriate, intonation, range).

Box 3.2: Voice clinic questionnaire

VOICE PATIENT QUESTIONNAIRE

Date: __/__/__

Occupation / Previous occupation:

Married / Single / Widowed / Divorced

Your voice problems

How long have you had a voice problem? ____________________

What are the main problems with your voice? ____________________

Does your voice problem come and go? ____________________

What time of day is it at its worst? ____________________

Describe how your voice sounds: ____________________

Describe how your throat feels: ____________________

Do you recognize anything that makes the problem worse? ____________________

Do you recognize anything that makes the problem better? ____________________

Do you find stressful situations make your voice worse? Yes / No

Have you had voice therapy / singing lessons before? Yes / No

Demands on your voice

How often do you use your voice
1. at work? ____________
2. at home? ____________
3. socially / hobbies? ______

Do you need to shout / speak with a very loud volume? Yes / No

Looking after your voice

How much do you drink per day
1. tea? ____________
2. coffee? ____________
3. water? ____________

How much alcohol do you drink per week?

Do you smoke? Yes / No   If yes, how much? ________

Do you have acid indigestion / heartburn? Yes / No

Do you suffer from or take medicines for (please circle):

hayfever	Yes / No	hormone replacement	Yes / No
blocked nose / catarrh	Yes / No	anxiety / depression	Yes / No
asthma	Yes / No	hearing problems / aids	Yes / No
cough	Yes / No	heartburn / hiatus hernia	Yes / No
neck / shoulder problems	Yes / No	swallowing problems	Yes / No
radiotherapy	Yes / No	thyroid problems	Yes / No

Reflux Symptom Index (RS)

Within the last MONTH, how did the following problems affect you?

(0 = No problem; 5 = Severe problem)

1. Hoarseness or problem with voice	0	1	2	3	4	5
2. Clearing your throat	0	1	2	3	4	5
3. Excess throat mucous or postnasal drip	0	1	2	3	4	5
4. Difficulty swallowing food, liquid, or pills	0	1	2	3	4	5
5. Coughing after you ate or after lying down	0	1	2	3	4	5
6. Breathing difficulties or choking episodes	0	1	2	3	4	5
7. Troublesome or annoying cough	0	1	2	3	4	5
8. Something sticking in throat or lump in throat	0	1	2	3	4	5
9. Heartburn, chest pain, indigestion	0	1	2	3	4	5

Voice-related quality of life

1 = None, not a problem 2 = A small amount 3 = A moderate (medium) amount
4 = A lot 5 = Problem is 'as bad as it can be'

Because of my voice:

1. I have trouble speaking loudly or being heard in noisy situations	0	1	2	3	4	5
2. I run out of air and need to take frequent breaths when talking	0	1	2	3	4	5
3. I sometimes do not know what will come out when I begin speaking	0	1	2	3	4	5
4. I am sometimes anxious or frustrated	0	1	2	3	4	5
5. I sometimes get depressed	0	1	2	3	4	5
6. I have trouble using the telephone	0	1	2	3	4	5
7. I have trouble doing my job or practicing my profession	0	1	2	3	4	5
8. I avoid going out socially	0	1	2	3	4	5
9. I have to repeat myself to be understood	0	1	2	3	4	5
10. I have become less outgoing	0	1	2	3	4	5

A widely used psychoacoustic measurement system is GRBAS (grade, roughness, breathiness, asthenia, and strain). Widely referenced in the literature, it can be easily taught, is quick to complete, and has good inter and intra rater reliability. It is, however, limited in sensitivity for describing some features such and consistency and smaller steps in the severity rating scale. Other subjective voice rating scales include Cape-V, Vocal Profile Analysis Protocol, GRBASI, and Voice Profile Analysis. The authors recommend further reading for more detailed information beyond the scope of this chapter.

It is the psychoacoustic features of voice that a specialist in voice disorders can be familiar with and can offer their expertise on in the operative theatre during framework surgery. Other objective measures can be used to assess and guide decision-making, as mentioned below, such as Peak Direct Subglottic Pressure (PDSGP). In the authors' practice the following voice tests are used in theatre (Figure 3.1):

1. Maximum Phonation Time (MPT) on /ee/ seconds;
2. MPT on a high pitch;
3. MPT on a low pitch;
4. glide upwards and down; and
5. number the patient can count to on one breath.

All voice clinicians need to be able to generally assess musculoskeletal and postural habits, observe breathing patterns at rest and in spoken/sung tasks, and make judgements regarding onward referral for issues outside of the therapist's or laryngologist's skills. Postural issues affecting the back, neck, shoulders, jaw, and pelvis will need to be examined. There are many good texts describing postural assessment and foundation for healthy voice production in the SLT and singing/voice coach literature. The authors also work closely with a specialist physiotherapy team.

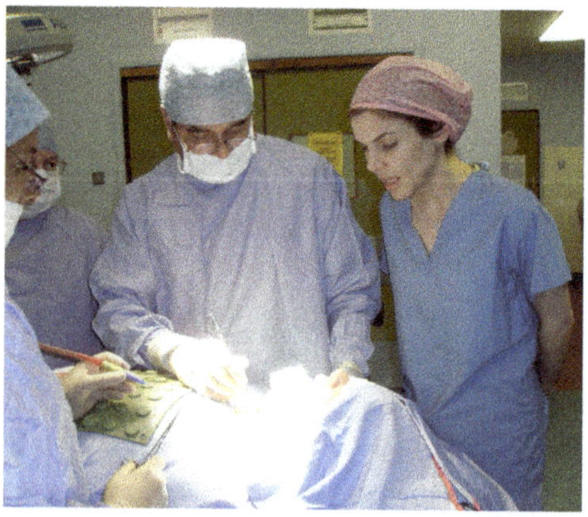

Figure 3.1: Voice assessment in theatre.

Many SLTs specializing in voice in the UK have additional skills in palpation assessment of laryngeal structural alignment and inappropriate muscle function within the larynx and neck.

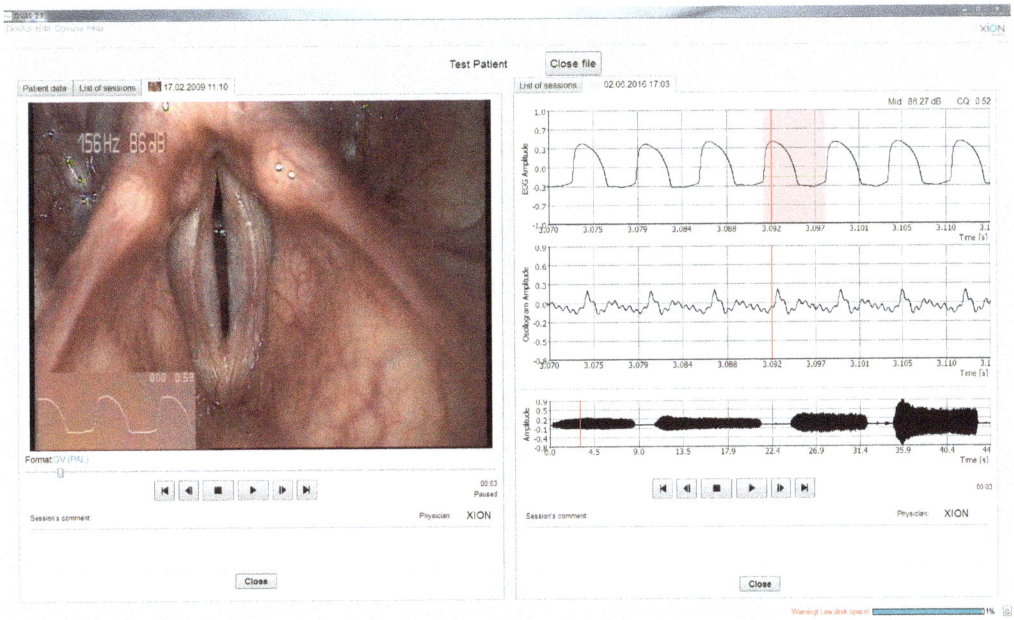

Figure 3.2: Electroglottographic assessment of mucosal wave.

Muscle tension and suboptimal alignment of laryngeal cartilages may be causing the voice disorder, but may also be the result of a laryngeal problem and reflect poor musculoskeletal compensation leading to hyperfunction.

Objective voice assessment

Essential assessment includes recording laryngeal physiology and vibratory patterns. Viewing the larynx and vocal function with digital flexible or rigid stroboscopy is described in detail in Chapter 4. Along with visual instrumental assessment, electroglottography (EGG) (Figure 3.2) provides useful additional information about the vibratory activity of the larynx.

One of the simplest, but still very useful, objective baseline measures is taking a good quality voice recording of a representative speech and voice sample. The sample speech and voice tasks can be carried out post-treatment and the recordings compared. Other frequently used techniques include aerodynamic measures, such as lung function tests; perturbation measures, such as jitter, shimmer, and noise to harmonic ratio; maximum phonation time (MPT); and s/z ratio. More detailed assessments are used in specialist research centres and will likely influence future practice. The authors suggest further reading along this volume for more information.

Intra-operative PDSGP is an objective measurement of vocal efficiency. It is being used more widely in awake procedures, in addition to standard perceptual subjective assessment by the surgeon and SLT in theatre. Current clinical investigations are aiming to validate the reliability of measuring PDSGP alongside subjective experienced clinical judgement and patient outcome for medialization laryngoplasty patients. Research and trials suggest the lower the PDSGP, the more appropriate the medialization for the patient and their perception of reduced vocal effort. Use of PDSGP is discussed in Chapter 7.

Swallowing assessment

The authors' practice is in the UK. SLTs' roles extend to the assessment and management of swallowing disorders. Many patients complain of issues associated with swallowing, including difficulty with liquids, solids, or both, food sticking to the throat, difficulty ingesting tablets, and globus sensation. Patients with neurological voice problems are at risk of swallowing difficulties due to changes in normal laryngeal movements during swallowing, changes in laryngeal sensation, and in many cases reduced airway protection during swallowing, resulting from poor glottic closure.

Patients undergoing framework surgery may have temporary changes to their swallowing function, coordination, and/or throat sensations. These patients will need SLT review and input to manage any difficulties during this post-operative period. Strategies such as FEES (flexible endoscopic evaluation of swallowing) or alternative feeding options (e.g., nasogastric (NG) tube feeding) is commented on in Chapter 8 on arytenoid rotation due to the invasive nature of the surgery which causessurgical swelling and bruising temporarily. As this is a procedure with known impact on swallowing, during the early recovery period swallowing assessment should be planned for pre- and post-operatively when the patient is ready to start eating. Other strategies available include modified diet consistencies and thickened fluids. It is also advisable to use validated swallowing related questionnaires, such as the Dysphagia Handicap Index (DHI), Eating Assessment Tool (EAT-10), and the M.D. Anderson Dysphagia Inventory (MDADI).

Further reading is recommended on this subject as a deeper discussion of the topic is beyond the remit of this book.

Voice therapy

Phonosurgery and voice therapy have similar purposes. Both are treatment options for voice disorders, both aim to change voice quality and phonatory capacity permanently, and both alter laryngeal physiology. Voice therapy is successful when the correct patients are selected and the appropriate choice of treatment (exercises/functional change) is delivered. Often, voice therapy is chosen as a conservative first line of treatment to buy time before surgery is undertaken, but this is not always a clinically appropriate intervention.

Sequence of events from client selection to post-surgical management

Patient selection

Prerequisites to voice therapy include:

- the capacity to change (physically and functionally);
- patient motivation;
- adequate hearing;
- the patience to allow time to change; and
- timing of treatment and commitment to practice.

Therapy targets and outcomes

Voice therapy techniques aim to:

- alter vocal misuse patterns (hyperfunction);
- resolve hypo adduction of vocal folds;
- minimize vocal abuse;
- optimize vocal stamina / endurance;
- optimize voice quality; and
- agree realistic goals for voice treatment outcome.

Evaluation of therapeutic outcome

Reevaluation throughout and at the end of treatment assists in determining perceived change of both the patient and clinician/s, objective change, and the patient's satisfaction. If the voice change in therapy or surgical treatment is dramatic, it is tempting to not complete post-treatment outcome assessments. It is helpful to continue with outcome measures should the patient re-present to the voice clinic with a return of voice difficulties. How will the clinician know whether the reappearance of voice problems is due to the same voice problem, or a new problem? Post- or peri-treatment reassessment is also helpful to provide feedback to patients who are dissatisfied with voice change. Being able to show a patient the improvements made, or not made, is helpful to determine the next management option, or to reconsider a particular chosen intervention.

When voice therapy is unsuccessful

Voice therapy is similar to surgery in that a lack of success from interventions can be multifactorial. It must be used appropriately to enable a successful outcome. Some issues that are not compatible with voice therapy interventions are:

- selecting unsuitable patients (physically and emotionally);
- using referrals simply due to other treatments failing ('when all else fails'); and
- prolonging therapy unnecessarily.

Voice therapy requires the patient to have adequate functional anatomy for therapeutic manoeuvres to succeed. (For example, an overly large phonatory gap is beyond even the most coordinated patient to use compensatory vocal fold adduction techniques to achieve vocal fold contact.) Diagnostic therapy can be useful in these cases when there is a discrepancy of opinion to demonstrate a more appropriate therapeutic pathway.

The voice therapy process is useful to allow time for patients to have a better understanding of what they are aiming for in treatment. This time can allow the clinician time to get to know the patient and their emotional wellbeing in more detail, and determine if onward referral is warranted as part of their management plan. Psychological issues can impact significantly on successful treatment outcomes.

Post-operative SLT advice and management.

In the authors' practice, the following is routine advice and follow up for patients undergoing laryngeal framework surgery. The sequence is tailored to the individual situation as appropriate.

Immediate post-operative advice for medialization surgery patients and voice therapy

On the day, patients are advised:

- they should not speak or where possible cough harshly for 48–72 hours;
- the laryngologist will check each patient post-operatively with the SLT;
- they should not eat or drink for two hours, or until the effects of the anaesthetic have worn off;
- they may find small amounts of blood in their saliva: this is not a cause for concern;
- their throat is likely to feel sore once the anaesthetic has worn off, and possibly for several days after the procedure, and they should take painkillers as required; and
- no special modification of diet is required, but softer foods may be more comfortable initially.

Some patients have reported a 'tugging' sensation in their throat when swallowing for a few days. In such instances, a slight chin tilt during the swallow and consuming softer foods can help. Arytenoid rotation and vocal fold lateralization patients will need more detailed swallowing assessment and follow up.

Voice use for the first week

Patients are advised that:

- it may be necessary to take the following week to two weeks off work and plan to avoid chairing meetings, telephone working, lecturing/teaching, etc., depending on their specific voice demands;
- the voice will sound different and sometimes will improve over the first one or two weeks;
- the voice/throat may feel different to use;
- they should use a quieter than normal conversational voice for first week and avoid athletic vocal behaviours such as singing or shouting for five weeks; appropriateness to start/restart voice therapy will be assessed at the first post-operative voice clinic review;
- they should try to reduce vocal effort levels as, now that glottic closure has been achieved, effortful laryngeal compensatory behaviours are no longer necessary; and

- staples/stitches on the skin of the neck are removed after one week if there are no issues with wound healing.

Telephone review at one week

- Therapist listens to voice quality and evaluates improvement in glottic closure and whether hyperfunctional compensatory behaviours are persisting or have resolved.
- GRBAS rating performed.
- Therapist asks patient's opinion on the improvement in voice quality, volume, vocal effort levels, comfort, and shortness of breath during speech and any changes positive or negative regarding swallowing.
- If the therapist and patient agree that the result is sub-optimal, a further telephone review is arranged and findings are discussed with the laryngologist prior to review in the voice clinic to determine the best management plan.

SLT management of sub-optimal outcomes

- All patients are followed up in the voice clinic 3–4 weeks post-operatively. All pre-operative vocal parameters are reassessed for outcome documentation and management planning.
- Many patients (60–70%) do not require further voice therapy after medialization.
- If the voice remains aesthenic or breathy post-laryngoplasty, it is likely that complete medialization has not been achieved, and a nasendoscopy may be beneficial to evaluate whether a top-up injection is more appropriate than voice therapy, or whether voice therapy techniques will be enough to optimize the outcome to a satisfactory level.
- If the voice has become 'tight', strained, or rough (when it had not previously been so), it may be that too much medialization has occurred, or there is surgical swelling present that is temporarily medializing the vocal folds. The fold then is too swollen to support a mucosal wave. This is best evaluated under endoscopy and is unlikely to respond to voice therapy. Good vocal hygiene is essential to enable best recovery of any post-surgical swelling. The patient will need to be advised that the voice will improve as the swelling resolves.

- If the voice was strained and rough prior to medialization and remains so afterwards, this may indicate that the patient is continuing to use the hyperfunctional supraglottic muscular compensation behaviours which had developed in response to the original glottal insufficiency (e.g. false cord constriction or anterior–posterior constriction). The patient may be continuing with these behaviours because the medialization was inadequate and glottic insufficiency persists, in which case a top-up injection may be necessary, or a combination of the improved post-injection vocal cord proximity with voice therapy, as described above, may be beneficial. Alternatively, medialization may be fully adequate but the patient may be struggling to let go of these hyperfunctional muscular habits.

Concluding remarks

The SLT is an essential member of the voice team in voice assessment, trial therapy, treating pre-operatively, supporting the ENT intra-operatively, supporting the voice patient initially post-operatively with advice and follow up, evaluation of treatment outcomes, and further voice therapy to complete the treatment process. For treatment to be successful, the voice must sound better, have improved stamina, and be produced more efficiently.

Treatment outcomes are most successful when required surgery is carried out skilfully at an appropriate time in the patient's treatment pathway, the patient is compliant with voice care, involved in their therapy, and fully aware of the intended benefits and limitations of the treatment being offered. Comprehensive voice assessment and therapy will enhance a patient's understanding of their treatment options, reduce recovery time, minimize complications, and improve voice outcomes.

Further reading

Abitbol JJ. 2006. *Odyssey of the Voice*. San Diego, CA: Plural Publishing.

Almohizea MI, Prasad VM, Fakhoury R, et al. 2016. Using peak direct subglottic pressure level as an objective measure during medialization thyroplasty: a prospective study. *Eur Arch Otorhinolaryngol* 273(9):2607–11. doi: 10.1007/s00405-016-4059-5.

Aronson AE. 1990. *Clinical Voice Disorders*, 3rd edn. New York, NY: Thieme.

ASHA Special Interest Division 3, Voice and Voice Disorders. 2003. *Consensus Auditory-Perceptual Evaluation of Voice (CAPE-V)*. Available from: http://www.asha.org/uploadedFiles/members/divs/D3CAPEVprocedures.pdf [Accessed November 2016].

Belafsky PC, Postma GN, Koufmann JA. 2002. Validity and reliability of the reflux symptom index (RSI). *J Voice* **16**(2):274–7.

Colton R and Casper J. 1990. *Understanding Voice Problems: A Physiological Perspective for Diagnosis and Treatment*. Sydney: Williams & Wilkins.

Costello D and Gibbins N. 2014. Evaluation of voice outcome and quality-of-life measures. In: *Otorhinolaryngology-Head & Neck Surgery Series: Laryngology*. Bhattacharyya A, Nerurkar NK (eds). Delhi: Thieme; 103–108.

Epstein R. 2014. Management of voice disorders: key principles of speech and language therapy. In: *Otorhinolaryngology-Head & Neck Surgery Series: Laryngology*. Bhattacharyya A, Nerurkar NK (eds). Delhi: Thieme; 155–160.

Ford CN and Bless DN (eds). 1991. *Phonosurgery: Assessment and Surgical Management of Voice Disorders*. New York, NY: Raven Press.

Harris T, Harris S, Rubin JS, Howard DM. 1998. *The Voice Clinic Handbook*. London: Whurr.

Hirano M. 1983. Clinical examination of voice. In: Arnold GE, Winckel F, Wyke BD (eds). *Disorders of Human Communication*, 5th edn. Vienna and New York, NY: Springer.

Hogikyan ND, Sethuraman G. 1999. Validation of an instrument to measure voice-related quality of life (V-RQOL). *J Voice* **13**:557–69.

Jacobson BH, et al. 1997. The Voice Handicap Index (VHI): development and validation. *Am J Speech Lang Pathol* **6**:66–70.

Jones SM. 2016. *Laryngeal Endoscopy & Voice Therapy: A Clinical Guide*. Oxford: Compton Publishing.

Mathieson L. 2007. Greene & Mathieson's *The Voice & Its Disorders*, 6 edn. London: Whurr.

McGlashan J and Fourcin A. 2008. Objective evaluation of the voice. In: *Scott-Brown's Otorhinolaryngology, Head and Neck Surgery*, 7th edn. Gleeson M, et al. (eds). London: Hodder Arnold; chapter 166.

Rubin JS, Sataloff RT, and Korovin G (eds). (2006) *The Diagnosis and Treatment of Voice Disorders*, 3rd edn. San Diego, CA: Plural Publishing.

Seidner W and Nawka T. 2014. *Aids to Voice Diagnostics: By Professionals for Professionals*. Berlin: Xion GmbH.

Shewell C. 2009. *Voice Work: Art and Science in Changing Voices*. Chichester: Wiley-Blackwell.

Wilson JA, et al. 2004. The Voice System Scale (VoiSS) and the Voice Handicap Index (VHI): a comparison of structure and content. *Clin Otolaryngol Allied Sci* **29**(2): 169–174.

4

Objective laryngeal assessment and principles of stroboscopy

Julian McGlashan

Introduction

Visual inspection of the laryngopharynx is a key element in the assessment of a patient presenting with hoarseness, throat symptoms, and swallowing difficulties to secondary care. In most ear, nose, throat (ENT) clinics today the examination is performed using a flexible endoscope passed through the nose using a constant light source. Alternative techniques include indirect laryngoscopy using a laryngeal mirror or a rigid endoscope inserted through the mouth. Using a stroboscopic light source provides additional information about the vibratory patterns of the vocal folds and is useful in detecting more subtle structural abnormalities. Stroboscopy has been shown to improve the diagnostic accuracy in up to 30% of cases when compared to the gold standard of a diagnostic microlaryngoscopy. It is really beneficial for clinicians interested in voice disorders to be able to use all of the above laryngeal examination techniques and have access to a stroboscopic stack system to tailor the examination to the patient and their voice problem.

Principles of stroboscopy

The vocal folds vibrate during phonation at rates faster than the eye can perceive. The oscillatory movement of the mucosa is known as the mucosal waves (Figure 4.1). When using a constant light source, details of the vibratory motion cannot be seen and the edges of the vocal folds appear blurred. A stroboscopic light source produces a series of bright flashes of light of brief duration (10 μs), which creates an illusion of 'freezing' the motion of the vibrating vocal folds. If the frequency of the flash of light is at the same frequency of vibration of the vocal folds then the same phase of the mucosal wave will be illuminated each time. Commonly, a slight delay is built in to the timing of the flash so that progressive phases of the mucosal wave are illuminated each time, i.e. out of phase. When each of these images are recorded and viewed at a standard video rate (25 frames per second) then the vocal folds appear to be vibrating in slow motion. This motion is only a representation of real vocal fold vibration, however, due to the time it takes to store the image on the charged coupled device (CCD) of the camera. To see the real motion, images need to be captured at a rate of over 2000 frames per second. This can be used in practice using high-speed digital imaging.

Equipment

Indirect laryngoscopy

Indirect laryngoscopy involves placing a small angled mirror against the soft palate whilst holding the tongue with a dental napkin. Light from a headlamp or reflected from a head mirror is projected onto the vocal folds and the examiner views the images. It used to be the mainstay of laryngeal examination in ENT clinics, but has largely been superseded by flexible transnasal laryngoscopy. It remains, however, a simple cost-effective method of screening of structural pathology of the larynx, hypopharynx, and tongue base, and abnormalities of vocal cord adduction and abduction. It has been reported that 10% of patients are unable to tolerate the procedure, and in up to 50% the view is incomplete.

Flexible transnasal laryngoscopy

Flexible fibreoptic endoscopes (outer diameter (OD) 3.6 mm) are the most widely used instruments for assessing the structure, function, and presence of pathology in the laryngopharynx. As it is passed through the nose and nasal cavity, post-nasal space and palatal function can also be checked. Fibreoptic endoscopes are mostly used with a constant light source (halogen or xenon) with images viewed directly through the eyepiece or on a monitor via a CCD

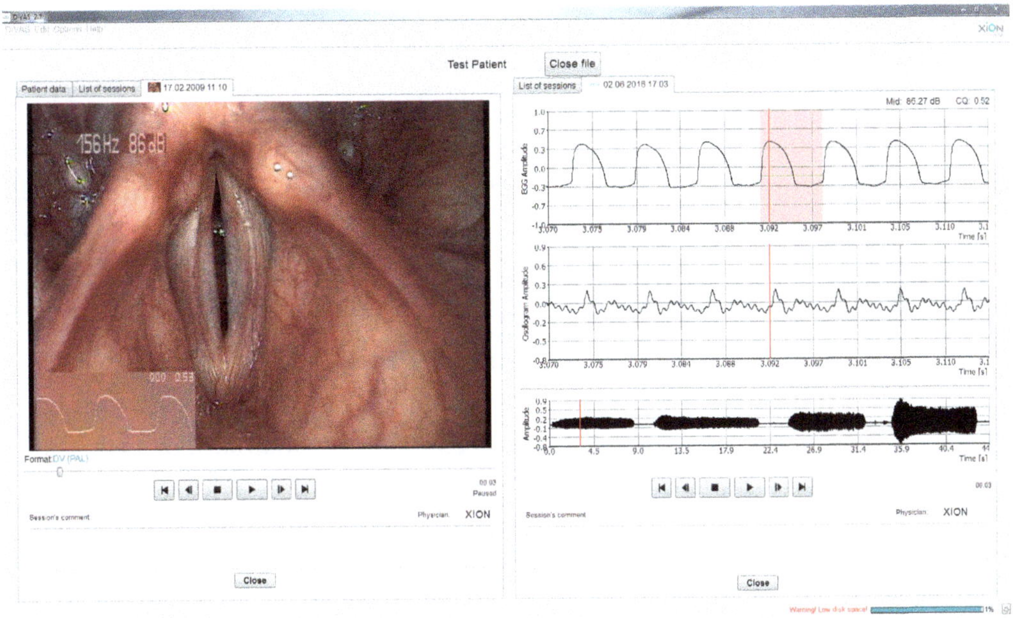

Figure 4.1: Electroglottograph demonstrating the mucosal wave. Image courtesy of Xion.

camera attached with a lens coupler to the eyepiece. Obtaining good quality video and stroboscopic images is difficult with this setup. This is due to the malalignment of the pixels on the CCD chip and the ends of the optical fibres, which often results in a slightly unfocused image or a Moiré fringe effect. They are also not primarily designed to be used with poorer illumination from the stroboscopic light, resulting in dark images.

Next generation videoscopes (OD 2.9–3.9 mm) have a CCD chip built into their distal end and give very good quality, magnified video images (Figure 4.2). They can be used with a stroboscopic light source. Even better quality images can be obtained with high definition (HD) endoscopes, but they have a wider diameter (3.9–5.5 mm) and cannot always be passed through the nasal cavity. The main drawback which prevents the widespread of use of videoscopes is that they cost at least twice that of a fibreoptic scope and require a

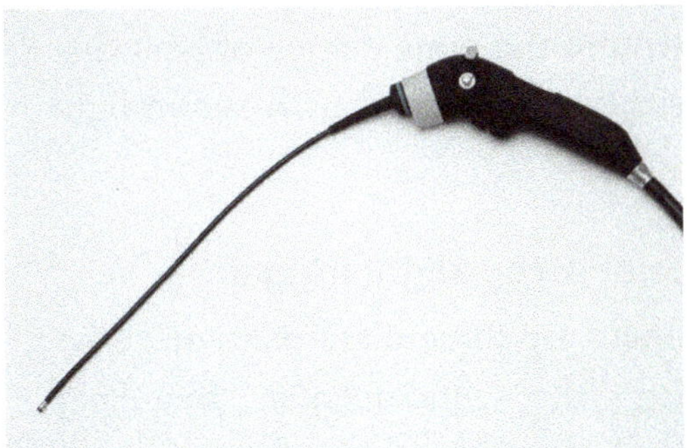

Figure 4.2: Xion flexible digital videoscope.

camera controlled unit, digital recording, and display device, although they can be cost effective in larger laryngology practices

Some models of flexible laryngoscopes have a working channel, which accommodates small biopsy forceps, laser fibres, and suction, allowing procedures to be performed in an outpatient setting where previously they would have to be performed in the operating theatre.

Rigid transoral laryngoscopy

Rigid endoscopes (Figure 4.3) consist of a series of optical rod lenses with a prism at their distal end (70° or 90°) allowing an angled view of the laryngopharynx. They are mostly used with a lens coupler and standard, or HD, CCD camera. The superior quality optics, particularly when used with a magnifying zoom lens coupler, enables them to be used with a high-speed digital camera. They give the best quality images and detail of the vocal folds when used with a stroboscopic light source. They tend to be used mostly in voice clinics and tend to be less well tolerated than transnasal endoscopy in patients with a brisk gag reflex. As the tongue has to be held, there are limitations to laryngeal and vocal assessment.

Light sources

Traditional constant light sources use either halogen or xenon bulbs. Xenon bulbs can also be used in stroboscopic light sources as they can be turned on and off rapidly and for a very brief duration. With the development of light emitting diode (LED) technology it is possible to use such light sources as an alternative, as they can also be switched on and off very rapidly. LEDs are cheaper and less bulky and do not require the same degree of heat dissipation associated with xenon light sources.

Stroboscope light trigger

There are three main ways of deriving the fundamental frequency (F0) of voice in order to trigger the stroboscope, each with advantages and disadvantages. Traditionally,

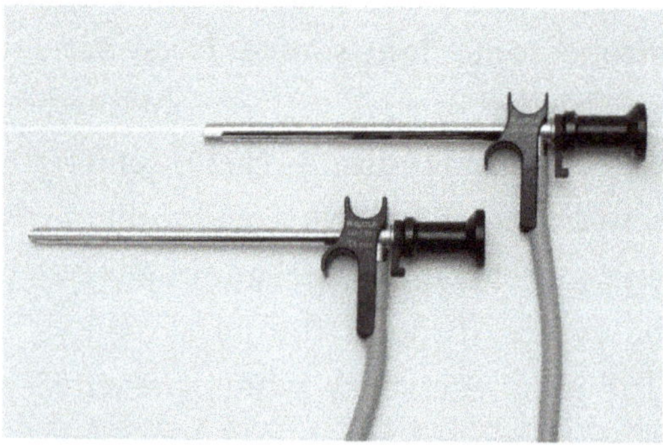

Figure 4.3: Rigid endoscopes by Storz. Upper scope is 90° angle and lower scope is 70°. Author image.

a microphone is placed near the mouth, sometimes mounted on the endoscope, to acquire the acoustic signal of the voice. A software algorithm is then used to calculate the fundamental frequency. This works well with good voices, but becomes less reliable with increasing dysphonia. Alternatively, a contact microphone can be placed on the skin of the neck over the larynx to pick up transmitted vibrations. A third alternative is to use an electroglottographic (EGG) signal derived from the change in conductance with vocal fold vibration between two electrodes placed over the thyroid lamina. Both the contact and EGG derived signals provide more reliable extraction of the fundamental frequency, except when the skin of the neck is thick.

Stack systems

In most voice clinics, where a stroboscope is used it comes as part of a package of equipment for ease of use (Figure 4.4). These 'stack systems' include a computer and monitor for digital recording and display of the laryngeal images. Such recordings are useful as a patient record for the comparison of changes over time, for later review of the images in slow motion and in more detail after they have been acquired, and for use in reassuring, informing, and educating patients.

Cameras and lens couplers

Rapid developments in camera technology mean that the new standard is high definition in medical grade cameras that can be attached to endoscopes. Zoom-lens couplers allow sharp focusing and variable magnification of the laryngeal images and, together with a rigid zooming scope and HD camera, can provide extraordinary detail of the vocal folds. The (×3) zoom facility enables variation in the image size from an overview of the laryngopharynx to a highly magnified image of the vocal folds. Fixed magnification lens cou-

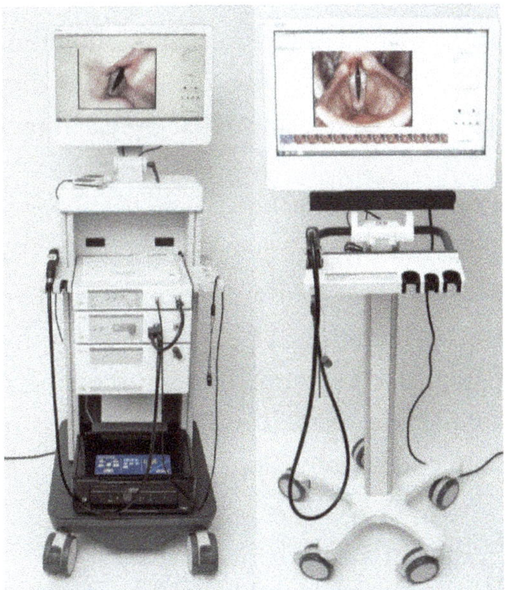

Figure 4.4: Stack systems – full stack on the left and portable stack on the right, both by Xion. Author image.

plers are an alternative and less expensive option but are a less versatile alternative, particularly if a camera system is used with both rigid and flexible endoscopes.

Digital recording

Video images are usually recorded directly onto a computer hard drive in a movie format, such as AVI or Mpeg files. Software facilities exist that allow compression and editing of the files to reduce their size for storage. Even though the price of data storage has reduced significantly over the last years, HD recording means that a 30 second, uncompressed AVI recording generates a 500 MB file. File compression means some loss of quality on playback, but this is of little significance in terms of image assessment.

Examination technique

A full explanation of the procedure should be given and verbal consent obtained.

Patient positioning and preparation

The patient should be encouraged to sit comfortably, leaning forward with their elbows resting on their knees, and with their neck slightly extended (Fig 4.6). It is important that their neck and shoulders are not hunched up and that they are as relaxed as possible. They should not turn their heads and try to look at the video monitor or close their eyes, as they need to focus on the examination task. They can be reassured that they can review the images later.

Examiner positioning

The examiner should stand or sit in front, slightly to one side of the patient at a level that is comfortable and which avoids unnecessary twisting and strain on the back and neck (Figure 4.5). The monitor should be positioned behind the patient's left shoulder for easy viewing. Many stroboscopic systems can be operated single-handed and utilize foot controls for video recording and/or stroboscopic light activation.

Endoscope set up

Prior to insertion of the endoscope, all the equipment should be tested to ensure it is set up and functioning correctly. White balancing and focusing where necessary is essential to record good quality images. Either a small amount of the patient's saliva (from the lateral tongue mucosa – not the dorsal surface) or an anti-fog agent can be applied to the lens tip to stop misting.

Flexible nasoendoscopy

A lubricated flexible nasoendoscope is advanced gently through the most open nasal passage either along the floor of the nose or above and medial to the inferior turbinate, whichever is easiest and most comfortable for the patient. Many examiners do not routinely use decongestive and/or topical anaesthetic sprays, although there is more chance of reflex tearing of the ipsilateral eye without spray.

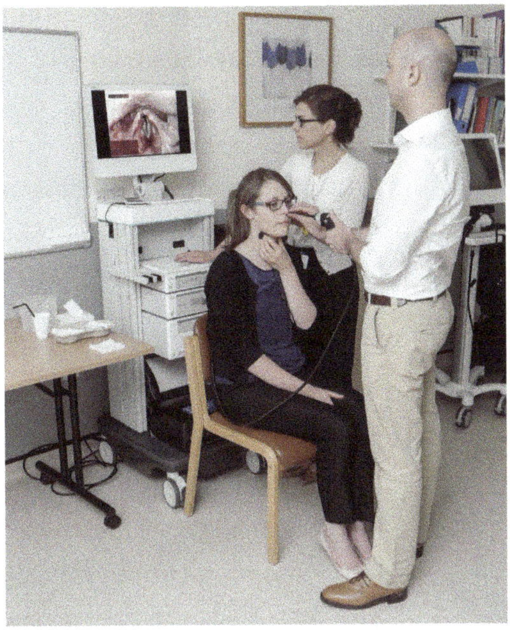

Figure 4.5: Position of patient and examiner for examination. Author image.

Rigid endoscopy

The tolerability of rigid endoscopy can be tested crudely by placing a tongue depressor on the dorsum of the tongue: if the patient allows the tongue to be depressed without significant resistance and gagging, then the rigid endoscope will usually be tolerated; if the patient gags on opening the mouth, then transnasal examination is usually necessary. The patient should lean forward and the tongue should be grasped gently with a dental napkin between the thumb inferiorly and index finger superiorly. The patient should be asked to take a deep breath in and make an 'ee' sound for as long as they are able. Once they have started to phonate, the endoscope is advanced towards the soft palate while avoiding rubbing the endoscope lens on the dorsum of the tongue, which causes soiling of the lens. While phonating, the patient is less likely to gag. If gagging is a problem, topical 1% lidocaine spray can help some patients, although it sometimes hinders others! If the back of the tongue rises, then asking the patient to say 'oo' can be tried.

Box 4.1: Examination protocol

1. **Examination: continuous light**
   a. Hypopharynx:
      lesions/pooling
      piriform fossae: openness, symmetry
   b. Larynx (sustained [i] 'ee' vowel):
      supraglottic gesture (MTD pattern)
      overall shape
      arytenoid position
      ventricular bands
      laryngeal rotation
      dystonic activity
   Physical condition of the larynx
      posterior glottis: erythema, obliqueness
      vocal folds: leukoplakia, lesions, dryness/mucus, inflammation
   Vocal fold opening/closing: repeated 'ee'
      abduction
      adduction
      glottal shape
      breathing
2. **Examination: stroboscopic light** (sustained [i] 'ee' vowel)
   Stroboscopy procedure:
      comfortable pitch and loudness
      high pitch
      low pitch
      increased loudness
   Observe:
      mucosal waves
         amplitude
         phase symmetry/lag
         localized inhibition/stiffness
      glottal gap: shape
      regularity
      effect of lesion on wave

3. **Indications for flexible endoscopic examination:**
   - Rigid endoscope not tolerated
   - Incomplete view with rigid endoscope
   - Examination of whole upper aerodigestive tract required
   - Need to observe larynx and vocal fold movement during
     - opening/closure
     - non-phonatory tasks
       - coughing
     - speech
     - respiration
     - singing
       - problem frequencies
       - passagio
       - glides
     - inspiratory phonation
     - feedback/response to speech therapy exercises/manoeuvres

Alternative techniques

High-speed digital imaging

An alternative method to stroboscopy is to use a standard light source with a high-speed digital camera. The equipment is currently more expensive and it also requires more imaging processing than the recording of stroboscopic images. It has not been shown to improve diagnostic accuracy over stroboscopy in most cases, but may play a part in the assessment of patients with severe dysphonia.

Diagnostic microlaryngoscopy

Sometimes, even with the best optical and stroboscopic equipment, it is not possible to differentiate between different subtle structural abnormalities such as sulcus vocalis, mucosal bridges, and particularly a combination of the two. In addition, deep intracordal cysts may only be apparent after a diagnostic microlaryngoscopy and cordotomy. Infiltrative conditions, such as amyloid, may be suspected but may only become apparent at operation. When there is diagnostic uncertainty in the presence of an impaired mucosal wave or chronic inflammation then diagnostic microlaryngoscopy +/-cordotomy is indicated.

Special considerations

Children

Paediatric fibreoptic and flexible video endoscopes (2.9 mm outer diameter) are now available. Children as young as five are able to tolerate a rigid examination, particularly with the smaller diameter (8 mm) 70° scope. They need careful direction but images can be obtained in approximately 50% of cases. Sometimes only a few frames can be recorded, but quality of the images is far superior with the flexible endoscope, particularly when used with a camera attached to the eyepiece.

Singers

Rigid endoscopy is useful to exclude a mucosal lesion, but overall flexible endoscopy is more useful in assessing functional and technical problems in singers. The most benefit comes when a singing teacher is also present in the clinic.

Further reading

Barker M and Dort JC. 1991. Laryngeal examination: a comparison of mirror examination with a rigid lens system. *J Otolaryngol* **20**:100–3.

Hillman RE and Mehta DD. 2010. The science of stroboscopic imaging. In: *Laryngeal Evaluation: Indirect Laryngoscopy to High-speed Digital Imaging*. Kendall AA, Leonard JR (eds). New York, NY and Stuttgart: Thieme; pp. 101–9.

Hirano M. 1991. Examination of vocal fold vibration. In: *Clinical Examination of Voice*. Vienna and New York, NY: Springer; pp. 43–65.

Kendall KA. 2010. Clinical applications for high-speed laryngeal imaging. In: *Laryngeal Evaluation: Indirect Laryngoscopy to High-speed Digital Imaging*. Kendall AA, Leonard JR (eds). New York, NY and Stuttgart: Thieme; pp 271–80.

Mendelsohn AH, Remacle M, Courey MS et al. 2013. The diagnostic role of high-speed vocal fold vibratory imaging. *J Voice* **27**:627–31.

Monnery PM, Smith WK, Hinton AE. 2001. Laryngoscopy findings in outpatient notes: the accuracy of the recording of the side of the lesion. *Clin Otolaryngol Allied Sci* **26**:278–80.

Patel R, Dailey S, Bless D. 2008. Comparison of high-speed digital imaging with stroboscopy for laryngeal imaging of glottal disorders. *Ann Otol Rhinol Laryngol* **117**:413–24.

Woo P, Colton R, Casper J, Brewer D. 1991. Diagnostic value of stroboscopic examination in hoarse patients. *J Voice* **5**:231–8.

5

Anaesthetic considerations for laryngeal framework surgery

Navneet Narula and Alexander Philip

Laryngeal framework surgery (LFS) embraces the gamut of surgical procedures designed to improve phonation and voice quality in patients suffering from vocal cord pathologies due to a variety of causes. Surgical aspects of these procedures are discussed elsewhere in this publication. In this chapter, we will look at anaesthetic management of such patients.

Pre-operative considerations

It is important to be aware of the initial pathology affecting the vocal cord that has prompted the need for the surgery as these medical and surgical issues are relevant to the anaesthetic planning. These may be classified into surgical and non surgical causes including idiopathic (Table 5.1).

Table 5.1: Surgical and non-surgical considerations affecting anaesthesia planning.

Surgical	**Carcinomas**
Thyroidectomy	Oesophageal
Pneumonectomy/lobectomy	Bronchogenic
Carotid endarterectomy	Carotid body
Other neck surgery	Parotid
Cardiac and aortic surgery	Other head and neck malignancies

In the surgical group, particular anaesthetic concerns would be:

1. Residual effects of the post-surgical state on the airway–vocal cord palsies, altered laryngeal and pharyngeal anatomy and sensation, airway narrowing and deviation.
2. Potential effects of:
   - chemotherapy – these include immunosuppression, liver, and haematological insufficiency and difficult venous access;
   - radiotherapy – these include immunosuppression and fibrosis of anterior neck structures and consequent potential for difficult airway; and
   - bronchogenic carcinomas – associated in particular with various paraneoplastic syndromes which must be looked for and considered in the anaesthetic management.

Suitability for laryngeal framework surgery is determined by the surgeon at initial assessment using a variety of tests. See Chapters 3 and 4.

Long-term smoking is a factor in most patients and its effect on cardiorespiratory systems should be borne in mind. Rarely, a patient may present with malnutrition in cases where dyspnoea and dysphagia complicate their disease state.

A baseline set of full blood count and a twelve-lead ECG should be considered for all patients presenting for LFS.

Peri-operative considerations

Issues to consider for the anaesthetist include:

1. The initial part of the surgery requires a relatively immobile surgical field with well suppressed airway reflexes.
2. The second part of the operation requires a cooperative, yet comfortable patient who can phonate on command to assess adequacy of surgical correction (important for thyroplasty procedures).
3. Sharing of the airway with the surgeon.
4. Typical theatre set-up (Figure 5.1).

Options for anaesthesia

Local anaesthetic infiltration alone

Local anaesthetic infiltration may be employed usefully for many types of LFS, but gaining access to the larynx will cause protective laryngeal reflexes to be activated, causing coughing, gagging, and potentially laryngospasm.

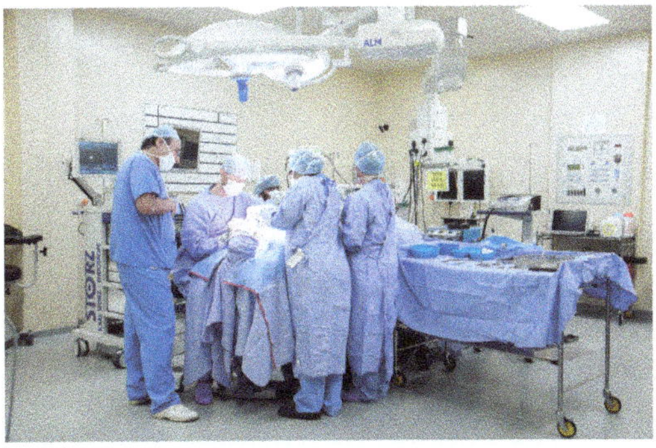

Figure 5.1: Operative set-up within theatres. Author image.

Intravenous sedation

Providing sedation helps to keep the patient calm, comfortable, and cooperative. Planes of sedation can be deepened or lightened depending on the phase of surgery; sedation levels can be increased when surgical access is obtained and lightened when patient cooperation for phonation is required. This achieves good results when combined with local anaesthetic infiltration of the surgical site. Standards of monitoring should be similar to when a general anaesthetic is employed.

Boluses of benzodiazepenes like midazolam, which can be reversed by its specific antagonist flumazenil when the patient needs to phonate, can be used. An intermittent bolusing technique does not result in a calm, comfortably sedated patient due to fluctuations in serum level of administered sedative.

A more preferable technique to enable a smooth anaesthetic and avoid swings in plasma level of sedation is to use a continuous infusion of sedation. A microprocessor controlled infusion pump that delivers intravenous sedation targeting a set plasma concentration depending on patient gender and body habitus, also known as target controlled infusion (TCI), provides optimum conditions for the surgeon.

The most popular drugs for this purpose are the anaesthetic induction agent Propofol (Box 5.1) and the ultra short acting opioid Remifentanil. These may be either administered separately or in combination.

Box 5.1: Dosage planning for a 70 kg male patient

Propofol TCI at 1 to 5 micrograms/ml (target plasma concentration) and Remifentanil TCI at 1 to 4 nanograms/ml (target plasma concentration) may be used. Dosages should be titrated to effect.

Advantages of a TCI technique include:

- rapid onset and offset of the effects of the anaesthetic;
- optimal surgical conditions-patient comfort and cooperation can both be secured by appropriate titration of the rate of infusion;
- lesser risk of nausea and vomiting;
- quicker turnaround of patients and discharge from hospital;
- excellent suppression of airway reflexes; and
- remifentanil will provide intense, short lasting peri-operative analgesia.

Dexmedetomidine is an alpha 2 adrenergic receptor agonist that has amnesic, sedative, anxiolytic, and analgesic properties. Current use is mainly limited to sedation in difficult cases on ICU but, elsewhere, use has been described for sedative indications where patient cooperation is indicated; for example, in awake fibreoptic intubation. Kitagawa et al. in a 2014 study showed that dexmeditomidine provided good suppression of airway reflexes and operating conditions in laryngeal framework surgery. Moreover it improved maximum phonation time post-operatively as a successful index in LFS compared to general anaesthesia. Experience with this agent for this purpose is currently limited in the UK.

Sedation levels can be monitored by clinical observation of oxygen saturation, respiratory rate, and patient response to surgical stimulation. A more objective measure can be obtained if bispectral index (BIS) monitoring is used. Electrodes attached to the forehead process EEG waves to measure the effects of sedatives on the brain. A numerical scale ranging from 0 (complete cortical silence) to 100 (awake) can be correlated to sedation endpoints. For LFS surgeries under TCI sedation with Propofol, a BIS score of 70 to 80 will ensure comfort for the patient, while also preventing hypoxia from airway obstruction.

General anaesthesia

Options for a general anaesthetic procedure include:

1. Using a microlaryngeal tube (MLT). This is a 5 or 5.5 mm internal diameter cuffed endotracheal tube that has a larger cuff and is longer than standard endotrachal tubes. As it has a thinner profile than standard endotracheal tubes, the surgeon is afforded better room to access laryngeal structures.

2. Using a laryngeal mask airway (LMA). This is a supraglottic airway device that has an inflatable cuff that sits above the glottic apparatus, allowing the surgeon access to the airway. A fibreoptic bronchoscope can be used via the LMA to view the vocal cords and glottis. The general anaesthetic can be maintained by a target controlled infusion (TCI) (Figure 5.1 and Figure 5.2).
3. Alternatively, the patient may be kept asleep on general anaesthetic for the initial part of the surgery, and woken up for the phonation stage. This can be best achieved by a TCI propofol infusion; the infusion rate may be appropriately lowered to enable a rapid, smooth wakening.

Advantages and disadvantages of general anaesthesia

Advantages of general anaesthesia:

1. Complete and effective suppression of laryngeal reflexes during manipulation of the laryngeal structures.
2. Better protection of the airway against aspiration.
3. Ability to provide intermittent positive pressure ventilation.

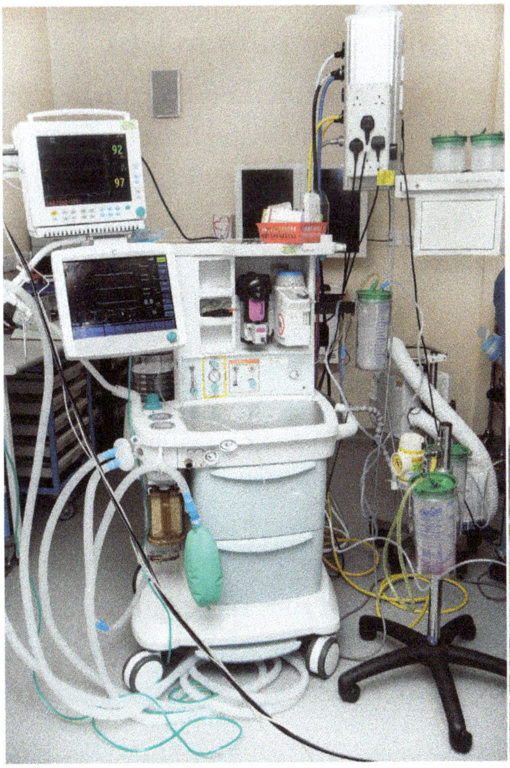

Figure 5.2: Anaesthetic machine. Author image.

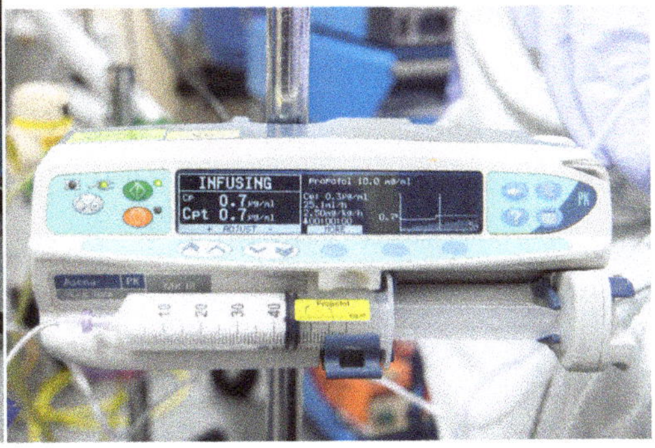

Figure 5.3: Target controlled infusion (TCI). Author image.

Disadvantages of general anaesthesia:

1. Patient cooperation is absent for phonation; this may affect outcome as surgeon loses a valuable feedback tool to alter surgical repair.
2. Airway device may cause alteration in laryngeal anatomy and make repair moredifficult.

Post-operative management

Close monitoring is required in the immediate post-operative phase to look for airway complications like bleeding and haemorrhage, and stridor due to the implant slipping. Simple oral analgesics, paracetamol, and non-steroidal anti-inflammatories (if not contraindicated) are usually sufficient. Voice rest is advised for 48 hours post-operatively – see Chapters 3, 6, and 7.

Early complications of LFS leading to airway compromise include

- airway bleeding;
- airway acute oedema and swelling;
- laryngeal trauma; and
- vocal fold haematoma.

Incidental surgery for patient with LFS implant in situ

There are very few reports in the literature about anaesthesia for a patient who presents with such an LFS implant in situ. Lin et al. published a retrospective review of post-medialization thyroplasty (MT) anaesthetics in a large teaching hospital of 219 post-MT patients, 74 of who had a subsequent general anaesthetic. Peri-operative airway incidents occurred in five patients. Three patients exhibited stridor in the operating or recovery room, which required nebulized adrenaline and intravenous steroids. One patient needed an urgent tracheotomy for severe stridor in the recovery area, and the fifth needed conversion for an LMA to an ET tube following persistent desaturation. They concluded that the peri-operative airway complications in post-MT patients needs to be taken seriously, and all involved staff need to be aware of the risks.

In an earlier review from 1999, the authors felt that post-intubation issues in such patients was minimal, based on their review of the anaesthetic charts of 17 patients who had a general anaesthetic post-MT. Nevertheless, the authors felt that the potential for airway compromise does exist, and suggest atraumatic intubation with a small endotracheal tube. Imaging of the neck to determine integrity of the device may be prudent.

Further reading

Friedlander P, Aygene E, Kraus DH. 1999. Prevention of airway complications in thyroplasty patients requiring endotracheal intubation. *Ann Otol Rhinol Laryngol* **108**(8):735–7.

Kitagawa Y, Kurashiki T, Fujii I, Inagaki Y. 2014. Monitored anaesthesia care with dexmedetomidine is superior to general anaesthesia for laryngeal framework surgery. *Eur J Anaesthesiol* **31**:14.

Lin HW, Bhattacharyya N. 2009. Incidence of perioperative airway complications in patients with previous medialization thyroplasty. *Laryngoscope* 119(4):675–8.

Morris S, Fleming JC, Child C, Harries M. 2012. Anaesthesia for thyroplasty. *J Anaesth Prac* **1**:17–18.

SECTION II: APPROXIMATION LARYNGOPLASTY

6

Type I thyroplasty: medialization with custom-made implant

Sharat Mohan, Smita Bangad, Kate Young, Owen Judd

Introduction

Medialization laryngoplasty (thyroplasty type I), the most commonly performed laryngeal framework surgery, has been practised for the last four decades. Prof. Nobuhiko Isshiki of the University of Kyoto, Japan, popularized this procedure and is generally regarded as the 'father' of laryngeal framework surgery (LFS). Initially it was performed mainly for symptomatic vocal fold paresis or paralysis, but over the years it has also been performed for other causes of glottic incompetence due to the following conditions:

- vocal fold atrophy (senile or congenital);
- sulcus;
- scarring of the vocal folds;
- post-cordectomy; and
- cocal fold immobility due to cricothyroid joint fixation.

This chapter is based on the principal author's experience of more than fifteen years with this particular technique, using custom-made silicone implants. Medialization thyroplasty using the Montgomery Thyroplasty Implant System (MTIS) is described in the next chapter.

Assessment and pre-operative work-up

History

Patients with a clear history of surgical trauma (iatrogenic) do not require extensive investigations. Symptoms – depending on the severity, chronicity, and history – should identify

- vocal impairment: hoarseness, breathiness, fatigue, and asthenia; and
- swallowing issues: dysphagia, globus, aspiration, and respiratory infections.

Examination

The range of examinations should include the following.

ENT and neck examination

- Examination of cranial nerves to look for neurological causes and co-existing pathology.
- Fibreoptic or rigid videolaryngostroboscopy with recording facilities: assess glottic gap, vocal fold vibratory patterns, and mucosal wave (see Chapter 3).
- Radiological assessment: CT scan from base skull to arch of aorta. Additionally, an MRI scan of skull base and brain may be helpful in high vagal lesions and other neurological conditions.
- Laryngeal electromyography (LEMG): helpful to differentiate between joint fixation and a surgical (iatrogenic) cause.

Voice assessment

The authors advise referring to the recommendations of the European Laryngology Society (ELS) Committee on Phoniatrics (see Chapter 3). These include:

- Voice Handicap Index (VHI);
- record of maximum phonation time (MPT);
- swallowing assessment: Dysphagia Handicap Index (DHI); and
- respiratory assessment: Cough Severity Index (CSI) and pulmonary function tests (PFTs).

Treatment options

Many patients respond well and do not require surgery. All are advised to undergo voice therapy, ideally over a six month period, before any surgery is contemplated.

However, if the patient is a professional voice user, and/or the voice therapist is of the opinion (after an appropriate number of sessions) that the likelihood of improvement is minimal, surgery may be considered earlier. A decision on early intervention will rely on the surgeon's experience and discretion.

The authors usually wait for six to nine months in cases of idiopathic vocal fold palsy if improvement with voice therapy is shown. An alternative treatment option could be a temporary vocal fold augmentation injection procedure before progression to a thyroplasty procedure if required at a later date.

Informed consent

The consent process and counselling should be tailored to suit individual patients and time taken to explain clearly the material risks and complications specific to them.

- Explain the benefits and risks of the procedure and explain the alternatives: surgery (e.g., injection vocal fold augmentation), or voice therapy alone.
- Provide printed and/or electronic media to reinforce this information and to remind patients of that which will have been discussed in their voice clinic appointment.
- Ensure easy access to the specialist speech and language therapist throughout the patient pathway.
- Discuss the type of anaesthetic (local vs. general). Reassure the patient that an anaesthetist will be present in theatre, even if the operation is done under local anaesthetic. The authors recommend target controlled infusion (TCI), as discussed in Chapter 5.
- Outline other peri- and post-operative issues that may occur. These include pain, bleeding, infection, scar at skin incision, airway compromise (leading to a possible tracheostomy), implant dislodgement, implant extrusion, change in voice, possibility of revision or top-up injection procedures, length of hospital stay, and ongoing care.
- Warn the patient and, where appropriate, family against any unrealistic expectations. In our words: 'If your voice is now two out of ten, we will aim to achieve six or seven out of ten. Please do not expect ten out of ten!' In one of our patient's words after successful surgery: 'In addition to having a stronger voice I can now string more words together without being out of breath!' (An improvement in MPT.)

Medialization thyroplasty procedure

Instrumentation

We would recommend using a standard thyroplasty operating set as shown in Figure 6.1.

Operative procedure

Step 1

- Position – supine, neck extended.
- Landmarks – superior thyroid notch, lower border of thyroid cartilage, upper border of cricoid cartilage, suprasternal notch, mid-point of chin (Figure 6.2).

Step 2

- Infiltration with 1% lidocaine (10 ml) + 0.5% bupivacaine with adrenaline 1:200,000 (10 ml) (see also Chapter 5 on anaesthesia). Infiltrate skin, subcutaneous tissue, muscles up to the cartilage (Figure 6.3).

Step 3

- Make a horizontal skin crease incision (approx. 5 cm) just above the lower border of the thyroid cartilage on the proposed side of the procedure, with the incision crossing the midline by about 1 cm (Figure 6.4).
- Divide subcutaneous tissue and platysma. Divide or retract the strap muscles to expose the thyroid cartilage adequately (Figures 6.5 and 6.6). (The lower border of the thyroid ala should be adequately exposed and delineated.)

Step 4

- Use two or three pronged mastoid retractors to expose the ala (Figure 6.7).
- Elevate the mucoperichondrium with Rosen's knife (first incision knife) in a U-shaped fashion (Figure 6.8).

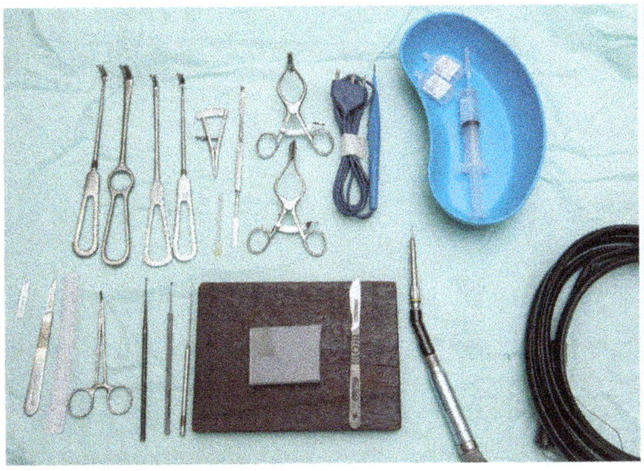

Figure 6.1: Instruments for thyroplasty in the principal author's centre. Author image.

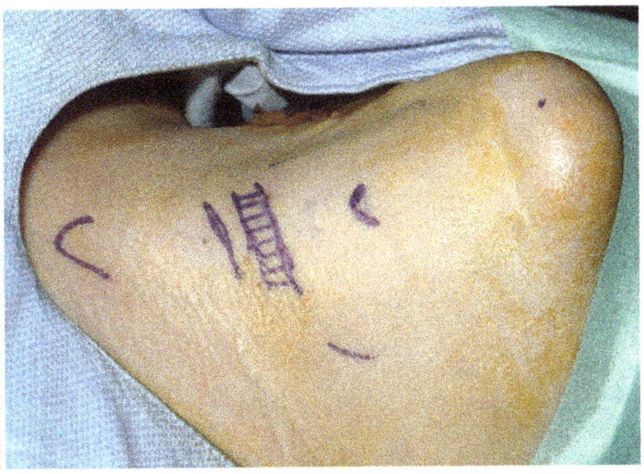

Figure 6.2: Landmarks. Note that the landmarks are drawn before infiltration of local anaesthetic (LA). Author image.

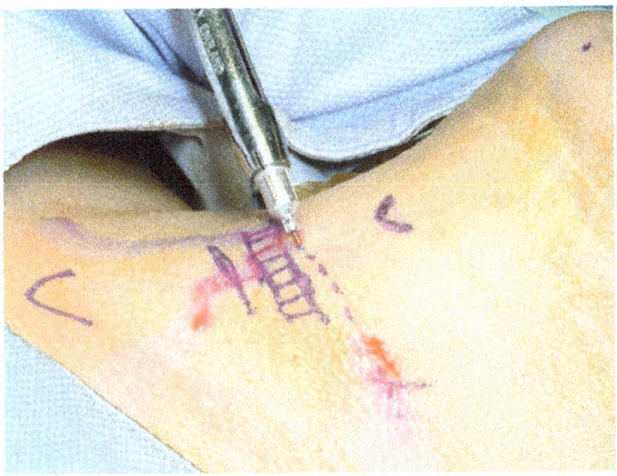

Figure 6.3: Infiltration of local anaesthetic. Author image.

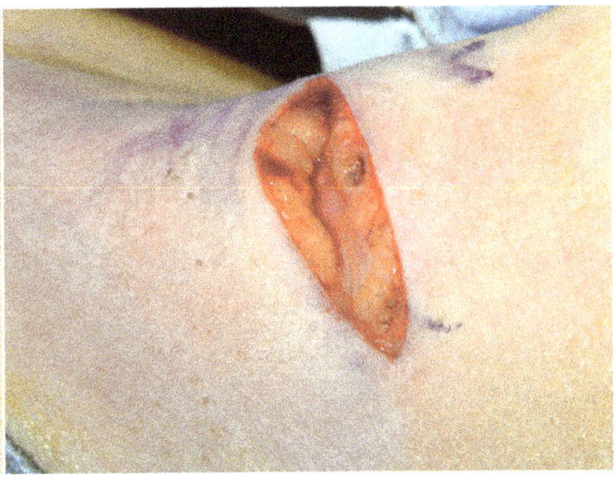

Figure 6.4: Skin incision. Author image.

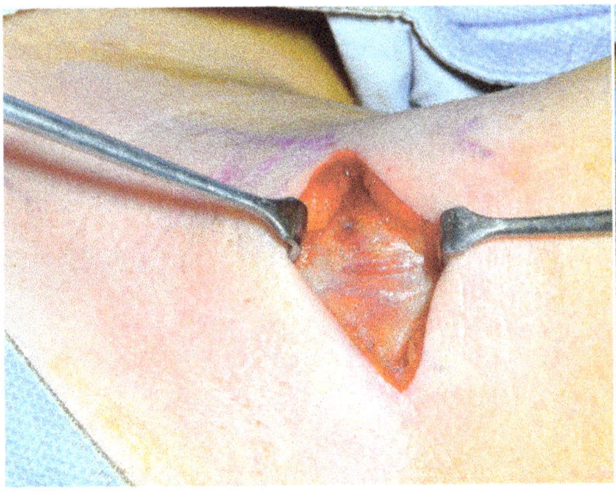

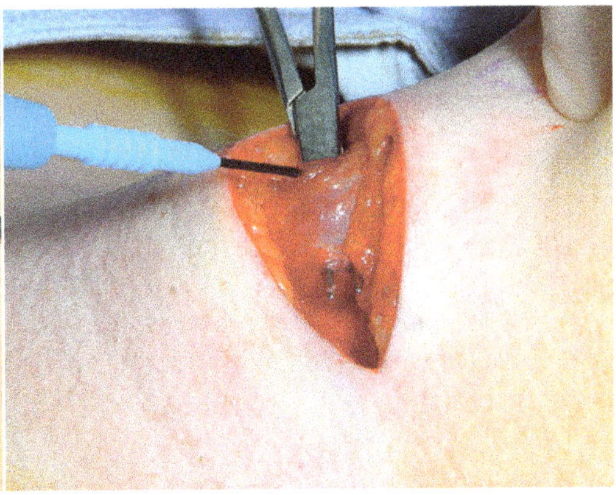

Figures 6.5 and 6.6: Identification and division of strap muscles. Author image.

Step 5

- Prepare the patient's nose with local anaesthetic spray or gel for flexible nasolaryngoscopy.

Step 6

- Using a calliper, measure the vertical height of the thyroid cartilage in the midline. This is the distance from the superior thyroid notch to the lower border. Mark the midpoint (MP) of this distance (measure from the lower border). This is point MP, and is the level of the anterior commissure in adults. Anterior commissure in a child's larynx is lower than the MP and the vocal folds are not horizontal but tilted anteriorly.

Step 7

- Using a 20-gauge needle, pierce the MP in a controlled screwing motion to pass through the cartilage to the anterior commissure (Figure 6.9). This will confirm the level of the vocal folds and is seen using a flexible nasolaryngoscope simultaneously. Care should be taken ***not*** to touch the posterior larynx, especially arytenoids, as this will stimulate the cough reflex and is also painful!

Step 8

Undertaking a vocal fold level check:

- The speech and language therapist (SLT) in our practice is present in theatre for the whole procedure and therefore is an un-scrubbed available clinician.
- A drape is placed across the patient, enabling the SLT to stand in close proximity in order to scope without risk of infection..
- The nasendoscope is passed and the vocal folds are viewed. If available, the scope is attached to a stack system in theatre. Once the vocal folds are seen, the needle passed prior by the surgeon (Step 7) is moved gently by the surgeon to indicate location (Figure 6.10).
- The needle position in relation to the upper edge of the vocal fold is confirmed (Figure 6.11).
- The scope is removed once the surgeon and SLT are satisfied with the assessment.

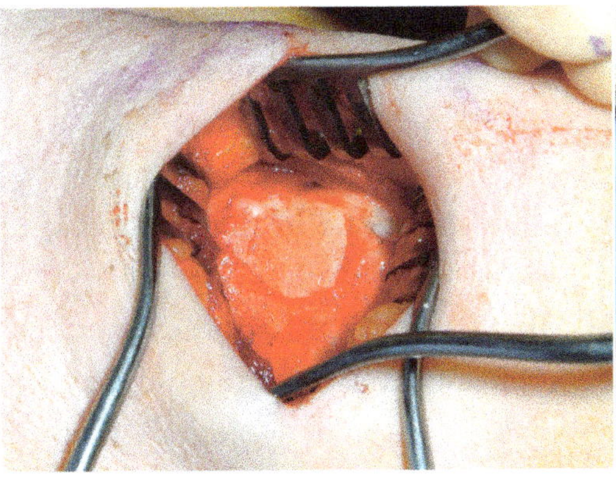

Figure 6.7: Exposure of thyroid ala. Author image.

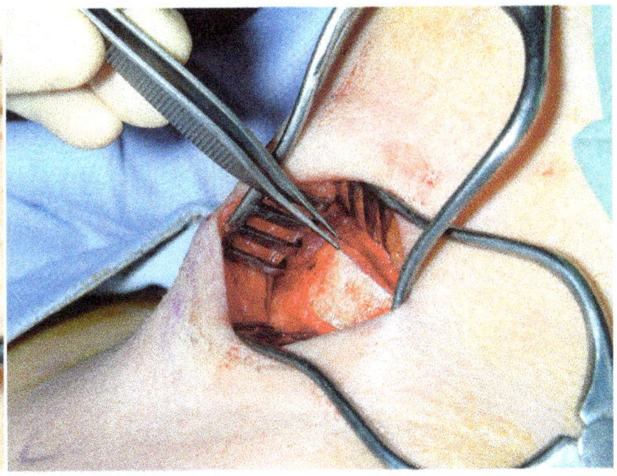

Figure 6.8: Mucoperichondrial flap. Author image.

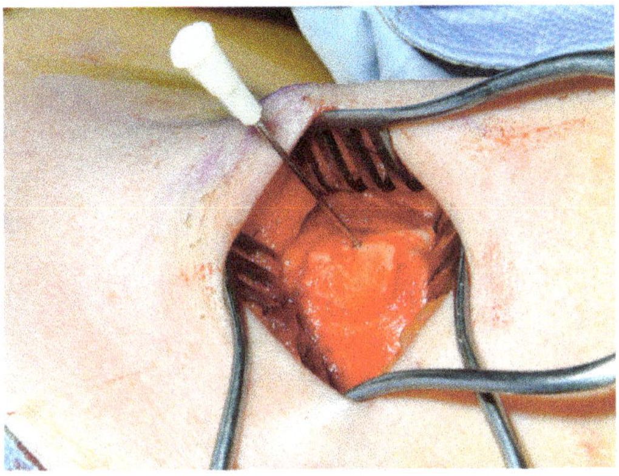

Figure 6.9: Needle confirming anterior commissure position. Author image.

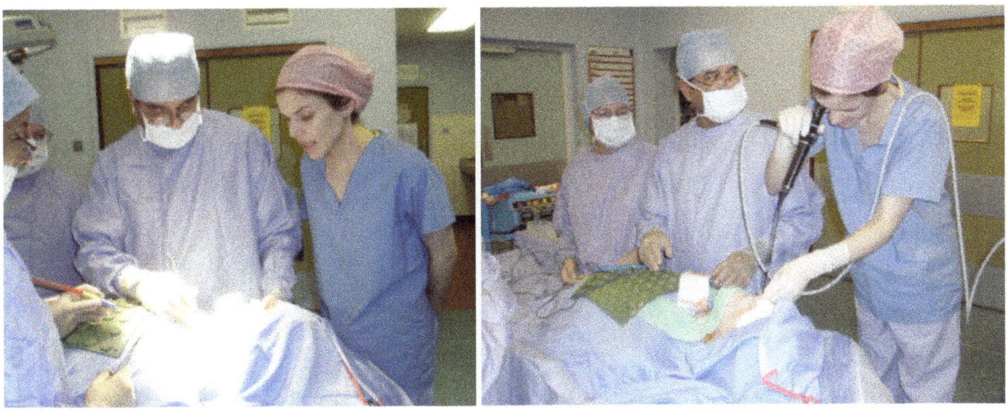

Figure 6.10: Assessment of voice (left) and nasendoscopy (right). Author image.

Step 9

- Mark the thyroplasty window as shown in Figure 6.12, using Table 6.1 as a guide to locating and creating the correct dimension.
- Connecting points A, B, C, and D (Table 6.1), mark the window using methylene blue or diathermy. The window should be in the lower half of the thyroid ala.
- The lower border of the window should be at least 3 mm from the lower border of the thyroid cartilage. This is to prevent fracture of the thyroid cartilage – especially in females and in patients who have undergone radiotherapy. Draw an imaginary line horizontally along the lower border of the thyroid ala when measuring the minimum 3 mm (ignore the lower thyroid tubercle).

Table 6.1: Dimensions of windows

Male			**Female**		
Point A	→	7 mm lateral to MP	Point A	→	5 mm lateral to MP
Point B	→	10 mm lateral to A	Point B	→	8 mm lateral to A
Point C	→	5 mm inferior to A	Point C	→	5 mm inferior to A
Point D	→	10 mm lateral to C	Point D	→	8 mm lateral to C
Window size is 10 mm × 5 mm			*Window size is 8 mm × 5 mm*		

Step 10

- Commence drilling out the window as follows:
  - Use a 1 mm cutting drill to carve out the window. Most cartilages are ossified and need a drill (Figures 6.13 and 6.14).
  - Soft cartilages can be carved out using a suitably sized blade on a Bard Parker knife.
  - Care should be taken when reaching the inner perichondrium to avoid perforation and possible extrusion, bleeding, or haemoatoma.
  - The cartilage window may be removed entirely, to expose the inner perichondrium.
- Alternatively, the following procedure can be adopted:
  - The cartilage window may be thinned out using a polishing drill to leave it intact in order to act as a platform for the implant (this method is helpful in prevention of implant extrusion into the airway, especially in females).

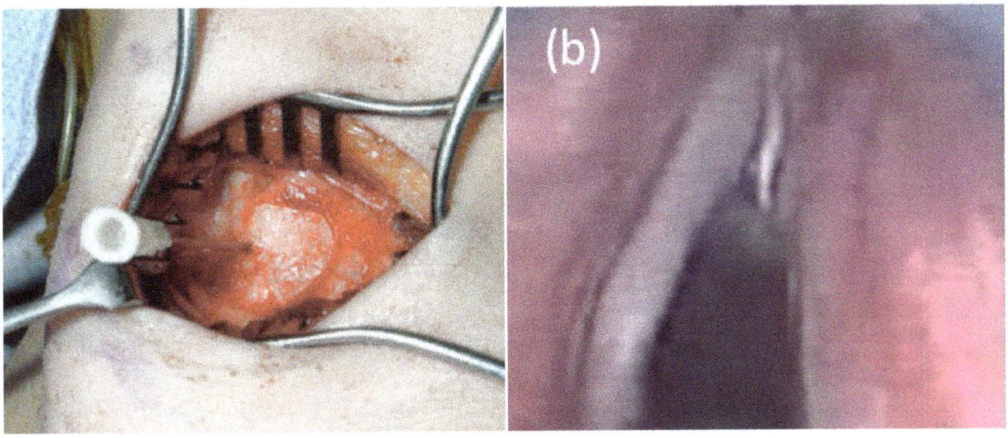

Figure 6.11: Needle confirming anterior commissure position externally (left) and internally (right). Author image.

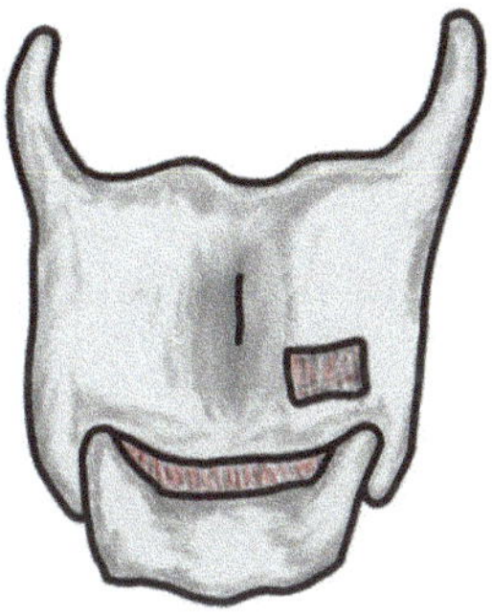

Figure 6.12: Position of window. Author image.

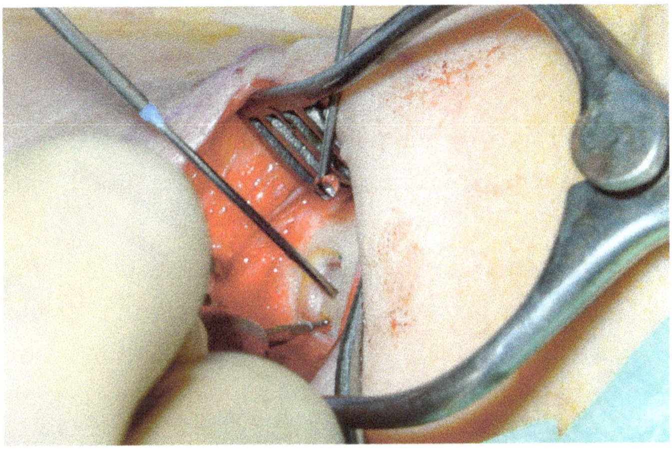

Figure 6.13: Drilling to carve out the window. Author image.

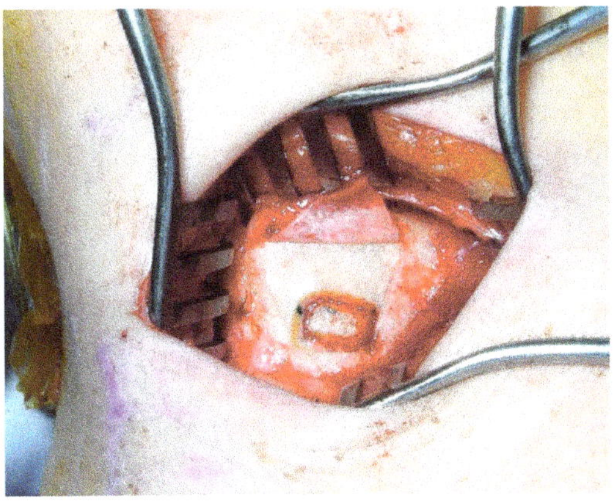

Figure 6.14: The completed window. Author image.

Step 11

- Use a blunt elevator (McDonald or Freer) to gently lift the inner perichondrium in all directions (Figure 6.15), taking care **not** to damage the laryngeal ventricle while undermining superiorly to prevent possible implant extrusion! See Figure 6.16.
- The patient and the anaesthetist are informed of the next step to make sure the patient is adequately awake and unsedated for voice monitoring.

Step 12

Ideally, this step should be carried out simultaneously, with a second surgeon completing Step 11. Begin carving the implant:

- Limit the time taken between drilling the window and placing the implant in order to minimize oedema. The assistance of a second surgeon/assistant can enable implant carving while the window is being drilled and save operative time.
- Using a No. 10 blade, cut out a segment from a Silastic® block (medium to hard silicon) measuring about 15 mm × 10 mm × 5 mm (Figure 6.17).
- Then shape an implant with a base, hood, anterior, and posterior flanges (Figure 6.18).
- The hood will have the same dimensions as the cartilage window.
- The anterior flange should be very thin – approx 1 mm – purely in order to keep the implant in place as medialization is not usually required anteriorly.
- The posterior flange can have a depth of 5 mm or more depending on the degree of medialization required.

Step 13

Checking the voice – strongly recommend the presence of the specialist speech and language therapist in theatre.

- Once the window is carved, use the back end of an elevator or a blunt instrument to medialize the vocal fold (Figure 6.19) in order to check the maximum improvement in voice achieved at various points of pressure in the window, as shown in Figure 6.20. As stated above, and as a general rule, the mid and posterior parts are the areas required to be medialized.
- During this step, place the patient's head in the neutral position, by removing the shoulder bolster or pillow.

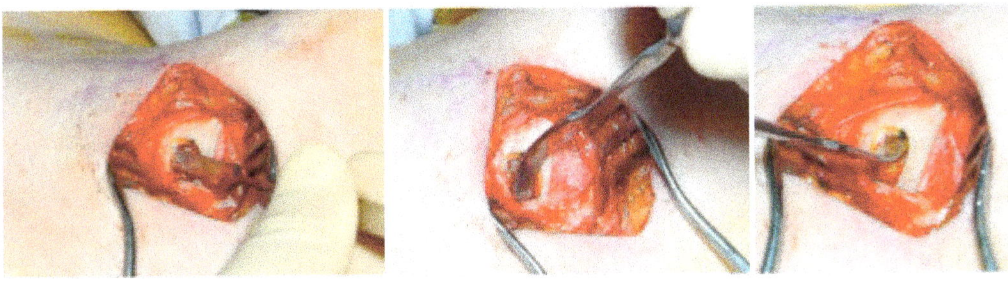

Figure 6.15: Undermining the inner perichondrium. Author image.

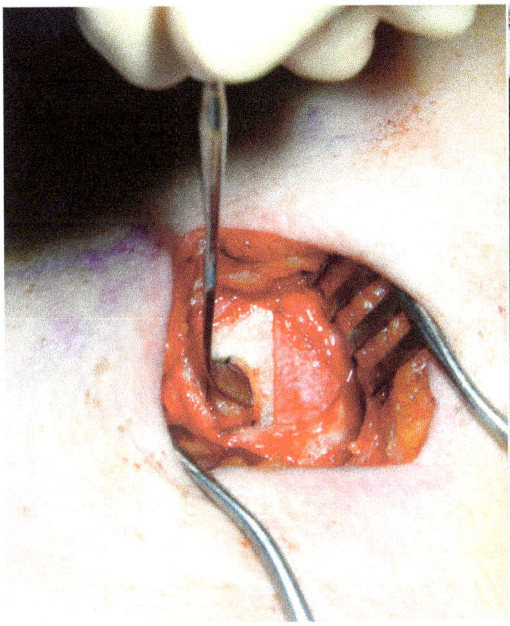

Figure 6.16: Careful superior undermining. Author image.

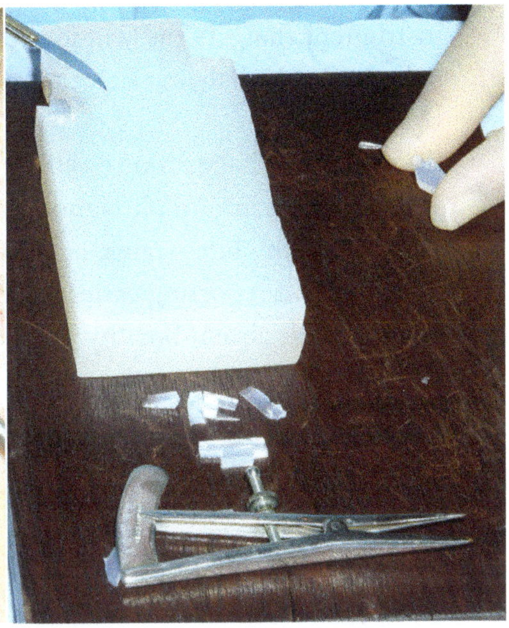

Figure 6.17: Carving the implant from a from a Silastic® block. Author image.

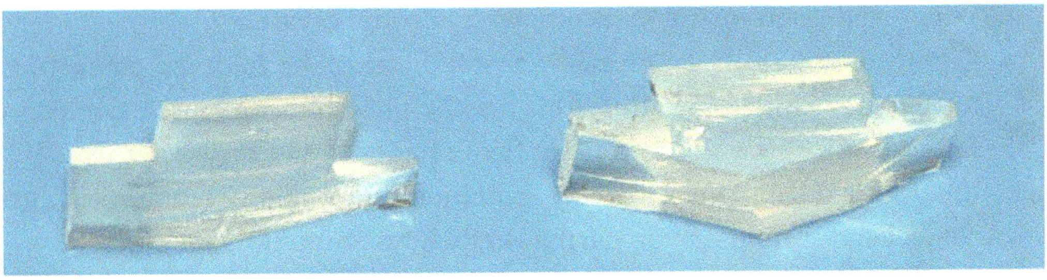

Figure 6.18: Final implants showing (a) base, (b) hood, (c) anterior flange, (d) posterior flange. Author image.

- Use adrenaline-soaked cotton wool balls in the window to minimize any ooze of blood, thus keeping the window dry.
- Moisten the patient's lips and mouth with a water-soaked sponge tip while checking the voice quality, as anaesthetic medications given may have caused some dehydration.

Step 14

While fitting the implant, undertake voice monitoring and trials as follows:

- While the surgeon pushes into the window with a blunt surgical instrument,that fits the window, trial the same voicing activities with the instrument medializing first the mid portion, then the back portion of the vocal fold.
- Successful medialization results in:
  - a longer maximum phonation time (MPT);
  - better pitch glides (range and voice quality);
  - the patient reporting easier phonation when asked;
  - reduced or absent breathy voice quality;
  - clearer voice quality; and
  - a 'voice' for patients who were aphonic pre-operatively.
- The SLT must work quickly and confidently, and be aware that the surgeon and the anaesthetist have the patient's medical interests to consider. The voice trial must be interrupted if a problem arises with the patient.
- Take time to make the patient comfortable and offer sips of water throughout voice testing.
- Ask the patient their experience of voicing during voice trials including their opinion of voice quality, volume, and ease of phonation achieved.
- Watch and listen for any difficulty with effortful breathing.
- Listen for any strain or 'pressed' voice indicating the folds are contacting for too long while phonating. This may be pre-operative muscle compensation due to the vocal fold palsy. Some patients find it difficult to avoid this acquired habit. Voice therapy techniques, encouraging gentle vocal fold contact and soft onsets for voicing, are helpful to use if this occurs.

Step 15

To undertake the implant insertion:

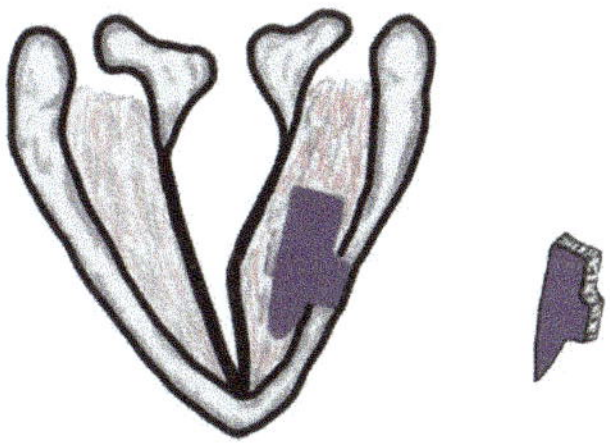

Figure 6.19: Implant in situ, medializing the left vocal fold. Author image.

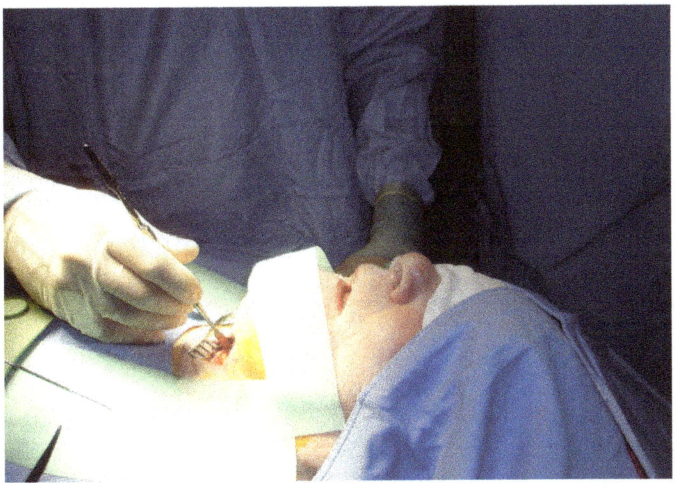

Figure 6.20: Voice testing during medialization. Author image.

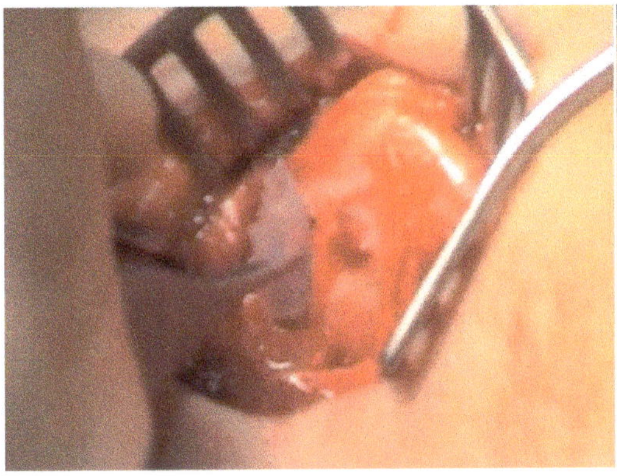

Figure 6.21: Inserting posterior flange of implant. Author image.

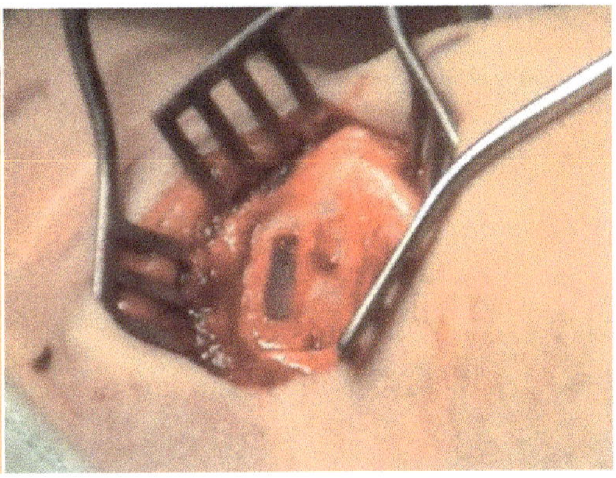

Figure 6.22: Implant in place. Author image.

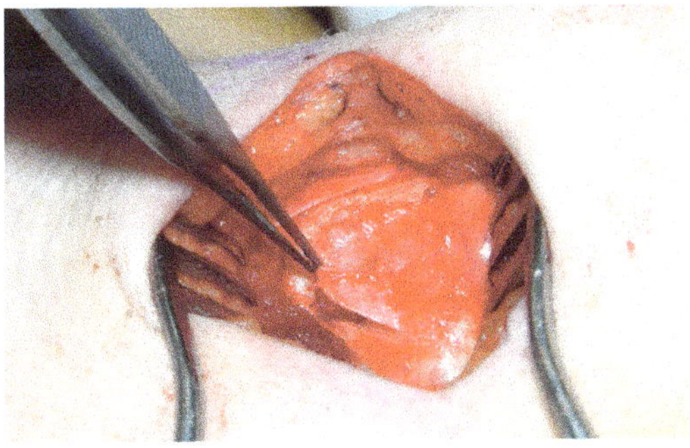

Figure 6.23: Replacing the perichondrial flap. Author image.

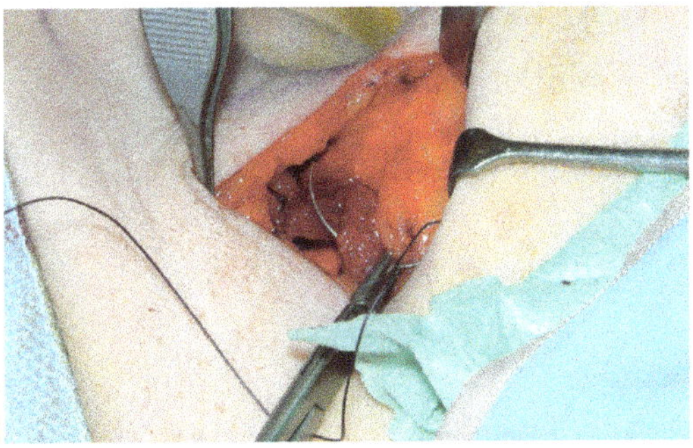

Figure 6.24: Closure. Author image.

- Hold the mid part of the implant firmly with a small artery forceps and place the posterior flange first (Figure 6.21). Then insert the anterior flange while an assistant helps 'slide in' the flange with a blunt instrument, such as a No.4 tympanic elevator or a McDonald elevator (Figure 6.22). To prevent breaking the implant during insertion, ***never*** use a sharp instrument.
- Check the patient's voice again with the implant in place. If the voice is too strained, it indicates that the implant is too large. The implant should be removed to shave off the excess and reinserted.
- Each implant is tailored to the degree of medialization required based on the phonatory gap assessed in the voice clinic and during voice testing intra-operatively.
- Vocal fold contact after implant insertion can be checked while on the table with nasendoscopy.
- Intra-operatively, dexamethasone 8–16 mg IV is given at the time of drilling the window and exposure of inner pericondrium.

Step 16

- The perichondrial flap is replaced but not sutured (Figure 6.23).

Step 17

- The wound is closed in layers and the strap muscles sutured back if divided (Figure 6.24). A drain is inserted and should be kept in place overnight (Figure 6.25).
- Intr-operative broad-spectrum antibiotics are given and should be continued for seven days post-operatively.
- Post-operatively, absolute voice rest is advised for 48 hours, followed by gentle voicing for two weeks.

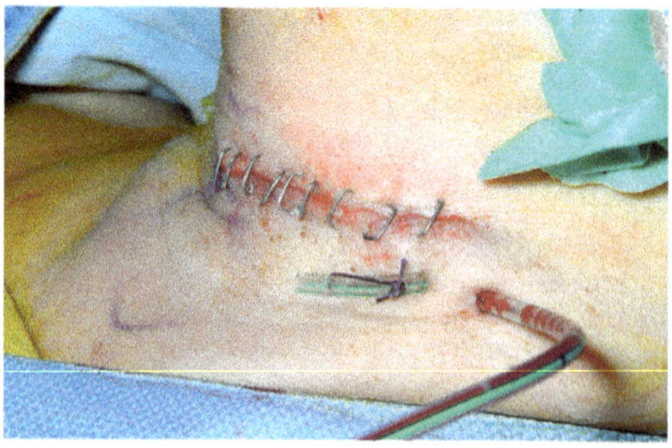

Figure 6.25: Applying a drain.

Post-operative voice care

- Patients are asked to have two days total voice rest and to avoid coughing and throat clearing to allow the implant to settle in position and be encapsulated. They may eat and drink normally but may prefer a soft diet for a few days.
- For voice use for the first week following total voice rest, patients are advised that:
  - it is necessary to take the following 1–2 weeks off work and to use a 'confidential voice' for 5–7 days, with frequent voice rests;
  - their voice will sound different for the first week, but there may be a temptation to use it as they will likely have had a disrupted voice for an extended period and feel motivated to use their 'new voice';
  - further, they should only speak at quiet or conversational volume for short periods of time for the first week;
  - voicing and swallowing may feel different to use: this will generally resolve and return to normal over the first week; and
  - the SLT will contact them by phone to discuss outcomes for voice and swallowing one week post-operatively (see Chapter 3).

Tips and pearls

- The upper border of the window should be at the same level as point MP.
- The window should be in the lower half of the thyroid ala.
- The lower border of the window should be at least 3 mm from the lower border of the thyroid cartilage.
- The anterior flange of the implant should be as thin as possible, otherwise it may result in a strained (pressed) voice.
- The posterior flange should ***not*** be too long, as it may impinge on the cricothyroid joint and hinder insertion. The shape of the implant can be modified accordingly.
- The time taken after the creation of the window to the insertion of the implant should be kept to a minimum to avoid oedema setting in. Oedema of the vocal folds can give an apparent improvement in voice quality and may result in under-correction. You may need to slightly over-correct if this is the case.

- The patient's head should be brought back to the neutral position while checking phonation, and the lips and tongue should be moistened to minimize the impact of anaesthetic medications.
- Beginners should select the neck carefully (a thin neck is ideal) and should practice carving the implant before the procedure.

Pitfalls

- The most common mistake is malposition of the implant within the supraglottis (Figure 6.26). Careful measuring and positioning of the window will avoid this.
- In patients with a short, fat neck (especially females), care should be taken not to create the window in the cricoid cartilage. The author has seen this happening.
- Excessive bleeding from the window edges may be controlled with quick bursts of diathermy and/or adrenaline soaked cotton wool balls or bone wax.

Conclusion

In the authors' experience, medialization thyroplasty is a very safe and effective procedure, especially if performed under local anaesthetic with target-controlled sedation. Other factors which can affect the outcome of surgery include the overall medical condition of the patient and the post-operative voice therapy sessions. The authors have noticed the optimum improvement in voice is at about 12 months post-operatively. All patients are followed up for a year before they are discharged.

Over a period of 15 years, the principal author has performed over 160 thyroplasty procedures, from which three patients had implant extrusion (Figure 6.27). All involved female patients and all were experienced prior to 2005, at which point we adopted the procedures described in this chapter. Since then, we have had no extrusions.

In patients with with dysphonia and aspiration as a result of advanced cancer, medialization thyroplasty under local anaesthetic offers substantial improvement in symptoms and hence improved quality of life.

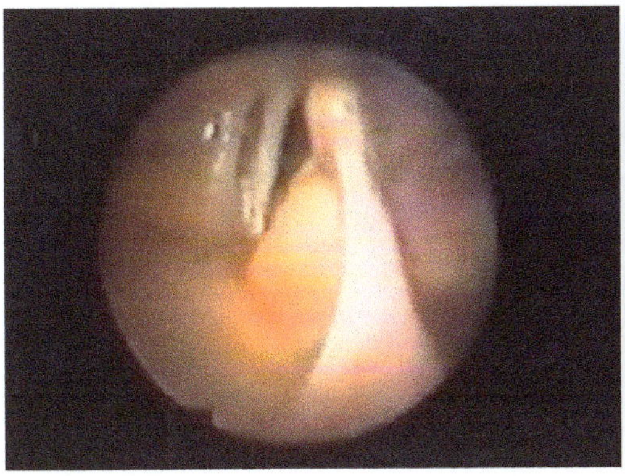

Figure 6.26: Implant in supraglottis. Author image.

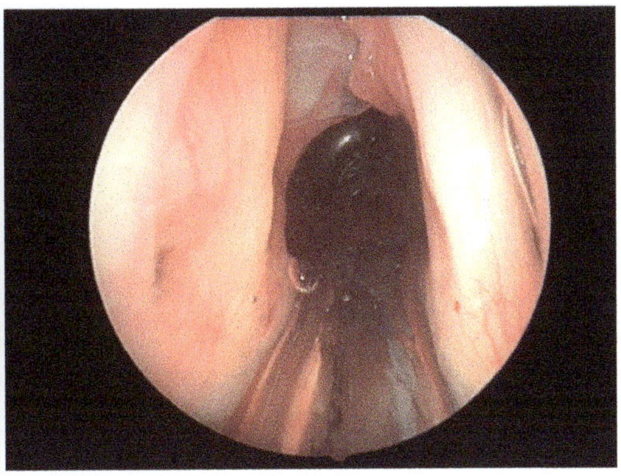

Figure 6.27: An example of an intralaryngeal implant extrusion. Author image.

Further reading

Carrau RL, Poy A, Eibling DE, et al. 1999. Laryngeal framework surgery for management of aspiration. *Head Neck* **21**(2):139–45.

Harries M and Gibbins N. 2014. Laryngeal framework surgery. In: *Otorhinolaryngology-Head & Neck Surgery Series: Laryngology*. Bhattacharyya A and Nerurkar NK (eds). Delhi: Theime 5:141–45.

Heuer R, Sataloff R, Emerich K, et al. (1997) Unilateral recurrent laryngeal nerve paralysis. The importance of preoperative voice therapy. *J Voice* **11**: 88–94.

Isshiki N et al. 2009. Progress in laryngeal framework surgery. *Acta Otol* **120**(2):120–7.

Isshiki N, Morita H, Okamura H, Hiramito M. 1974. Thyroplasty as a new phonosurgical technique. *Acta Otolaryngol* **78**:451–6.

Kartha S, Young K, Mohan S. 2011. Complications of medialisation of laryngoplasty. *Int J Phonosurgery & Laryngol* **1**(1):1–3.

Koufmann JA, Winston S. 1986. Laryngoplasty for vocal fold medialization, an alternative to Teflon. *Laryngoscope* **96**:726–31.

Stimpson P, Patel R, et al. 2001. Imaging strategies for investigating unilateral vocal fold palsy. *Clin Otol* 36(3):266–71.

Vinston KN, Zraick RI, Ragland FJ. 2010. Injection vs medialisation laryngoplasty for treatment of unilateral vocal fold paralysis. *Laryngoscope* **120**(9):1802–7.

7

Type I thyroplasty: medialization with Montgomery implant

Vyas Prasad and Marc Remacle

Conditions requiring medialization (type I) thyroplasty

Glottic incompetence caused by:

- unilateral vocal fold immobility – paralysis or fixation of cricoarytenoid joint;
- effects of endoscopic cordectomy – European Laryngological Society (ELS) Types IV–VI (usually);
- correction of scars and sulci; or
- congenital cordal atrophy (sulcus vergeture).

Assessment process, baseline measurements, and pre-operative work-up

History

Glottic incompetence presents in several ways depending on the cause, severity, chronology from time of onset and course (acute or chronic).

A thorough history should include identification of the following details:

- vocal impairment:
  - hoarseness,
  - breathiness,
  - voice fatigue,
  - voice weakness;

- issues with respiration:
  - dyspnoea,
  - exacerbation of asthma,
  - chest infections;
- aspiration:
  - cough,
  - choking;
- decreased exercise tolerance:
  - straining,
  - lifting,
  - valsalva;
- swallowing issues:
  - dysphagia,
  - symptoms of globus;
- emotional and social aspects:
  - quality of life issues;
- pain and discomfort when speaking, swallowing and breathing.

Clinical examination

In addition to a full ENT examination (including palpation of the neck and a lower cranial nerve assessment where necessary), all patients should have a fibre-optic nasendoscopy and laryngoscopy. We recommend videolaryngostroboscopy (VLS) with recording facilities – flexible or rigid – to provide a better assessment of the glottic gap, regularity of cord vibration, and mucosal wave.

Radiological and electrophysiological investigations

Patients who have had a clear history of trauma causing vocal cord injury, or surgery with iatrogenic involvement of the recurrent laryngeal nerves, do not require an exhaustive battery of investigations. However, where doubt exists as to whether the cause is due to joint fixation or paresis from neck surgery (e.g. thyroid, parathyroid, carotid, or cervical spine) with possible improvement, then a laryngeal electromyography (LEMG) can be helpful. The radiological examination of choice in idiopathic cases is a fine-cut contrast-enhanced CT scan from the skull base to the aortic arch. Gadolinium enhanced MRI scans of the skull base and brain may be helpful in high lesions of the vagus and other neurological conditions such as multiple sclerosis. In these rare cases, the superior laryngeal nerve is also affected, with corresponding loss of electrical activity on LEMG to the cricothyroid muscle.

Voice assessment

Vocal function is evaluated according to the protocol recommended by the Committee on Phoniatrics of the European Laryngological Society. This is a multidimensional set of minimal basic measurements suitable for all 'common' dysphonias. It consists of five different aspects:

- perception (grade, roughness, breathiness);
- videostroboscopy (closure, regularity, mucosal wave, and symmetry);
- acoustics (jitter, shimmer, F0 range, and softest intensity);
- aerodynamics (phonation quotient); and
- subjective rating (Voice Handicap Index –VHI, Visual Analogue Scale – VAS).

Swallow assessment

Despite the obvious vocal impediment resulting from glottic incompetence, especially from neurogenic causes, many patients complain of issues associated with swallowing, including difficulty with liquids, solids or both, food sticking to the throat, difficulty ingesting tablets and globus sensation. It is therefore worthwhile to investigate these issues further using both validated questionnaires such as the Dysphagia Handicap Index (DHI), Eating Assessment Tool (EAT-10) and the M.D. Anderson Dysphagia Inventory (MDADI). See Chapters 3 and 4.

Respiratory assessment

Patients also complain of cough, choking, worsening of asthma, and inability to clear secretions in their throat and chest. They may feel breathless when speaking or exercising and even at rest. Some clinicians use the Cough Severity Index (CSI) as a means of measuring the impact this has on patients. Pulmonary function tests and spirometry are rarely performed in this setting but, nevertheless, it is worthwhile to consider the impact on breathing due to glottic incompetence.

Treatment options and consent

The management of patients with glottic incompetence should be tailored according to the needs and expectations of the individual, the cause and course of the condition affecting the patient, and with the available expertise and equipment available to the clinician.

As is often the case in unilateral vocal fold impairment, many patients may present much later due to decompensation from a respiratory infection, or from greater demands placed from increased voice use, exercise or co-morbidities, such as asthma. As such, many patients may not require any surgical intervention. The following is a list of treatment options that may be used judiciously according to the needs and response of the patient, cause of the pathology, and availability of resources:

Non-surgical options

- Voice and swallow therapy.
- Chest physiotherapy.
- Dietary advice and modification.

Surgical options

- Endoscopic:
  - injectables:
    - long-lasting:
      - fat,
      - hydroxyapatite,
      - silicone;
    - temporary:
      - hyaluronic acid;
  - suture techniques (arytenoid adduction);
  - cartilage medialization.
- Open:
  - laryngeal framework surgery:
    - titanium implant (Friedrich's)2,
    - hydroxyapatite (VoCom)3,
    - silicone (Montgomery)4,5,
    - autologous cartilage;
  - arytenoid adduction;
  - arytenoidopexy.

Medialization thyroplasty type I (Isshiki) using the Montgomery® Thyroplasty Implant System (MTIS)

Consent

All patients undergoing surgery should be counselled appropriately about the benefits and risks of having the said procedure, not having it, and the pros and cons of it with the alternatives (surgical or medical) as well as the possibility of conservative management – which may potentially be the best option (informed consent). The type of anaesthesia, length of stay, peri-operative care, and post-operative course should be made known in simple and clear language to avoid unnecessary anxiety or misunderstanding. The multidisciplinary nature of treatment should be emphasized from the start, with good access to the voice pathologist throughout the patient pathway.

In type I thyroplasty using the MTIS, we counsel all patients on general operative risks, including that of local or general anaesthesia, pain, bleeding, and infection. Specific risks of the procedure include airway compromise and dyspnoea, posterior dislodgement, minor vocal fold haematoma, implant extrusion, breach after dissection into the laryngeal lumen, and worsening of voice early or late requiring re-insertion of a different sized implant. In cases where the patient has a fragile 'neocord' after ELS types IV or V cordectomy, an alternative material such as Gore-Tex® may be more suitable.

Operative procedure

Step 1 – Anaesthesia

Patients are given the option of having either a local anaesthetic with sedation and analgesia administered intravenously, or a general anaesthetic. Monitored anaesthetic care (MAC) during local anaesthesia is now more commonly performed in this setting. The benefits of local anaesthesia are that we can adjust the size of the Montgomery implant with the patient phonating (usually with the vowel /a/). We also measure the intra-operative Direct Peak Subglottic Pressure (DPSGP) using a trans-cricothyroid catheter that gives us an indication of the lowest subglottic pressures necessary to voice (Figure 7.1).

Local anaesthesia (LA)

- Intravenous opioid for pain control – remifentanyl.
- Intravenous benzodiazepine for amnesis and anxiolysis – midazolam.
- Intravenous short acting sedative and hypnotic – propofol.
- Anticholinergic – glycopyrrolate to reduce secretions.
- Local anaesthesia injection to operative site and trachea:
  - Lignocaine 1% with 1:200 000 adrenaline.
- Intravenous antibiotics pre-operatively.
- Intravenous corticosteroid pre-operatively.
- Oxygen administered via face mask.
- Cardiopulmonary monitoring.

General anaesthesia (GA)

- Laryngeal mask airway (LMA) preferred, over size 6 endotracheal tube.
- Transnasal fibreoptic videoendoscopy through LMA (Figure 7.2).
- Assessment of glottic closure and implant sizing.

Step 2 – Positioning

All patients are positioned supine with slight extension of the neck. In LA cases, the face is not covered to allow for interaction with the patient during assessment of phonation when deciding the implant size and measuring the DPSGP. A drape is placed on the patients chin and secured over two intravenous drip stands either side of the patient's head (Figure 7.3).

Step 3 – Specific equipment

The following is a list of equipment for insertion of the MTIS, as shown in Figure 7.4.

From left to right:

- Top: two window callipers (male – 9 mm and female – 7 mm).
- Bottom: two window outline instruments (male and female).
- Two curved traction hooks for thyroid cartilage.
- Two sharp hooks for cartilage elevation off thyroid window.
- Two duckbill elevators for inner perichondrium.
- One chisel elevator for inner perichondrium.
- Two implant inserters.

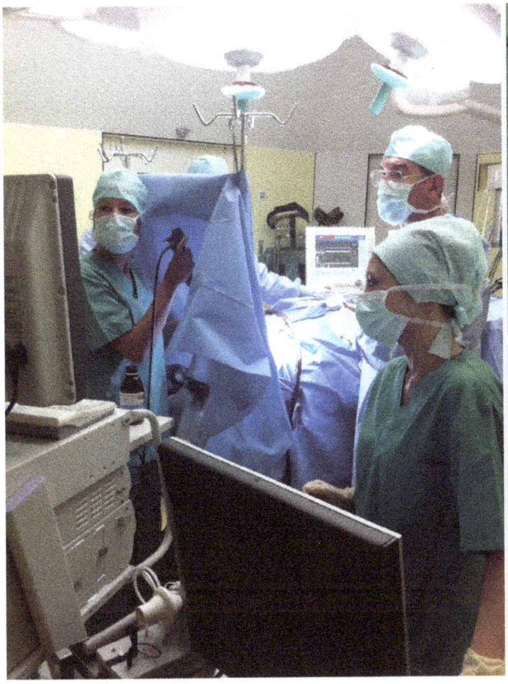

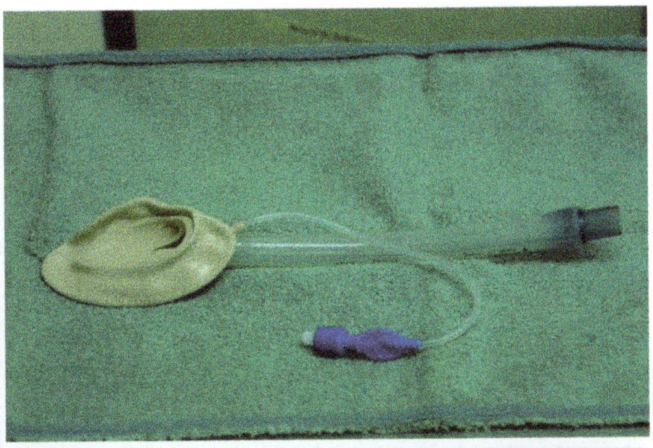

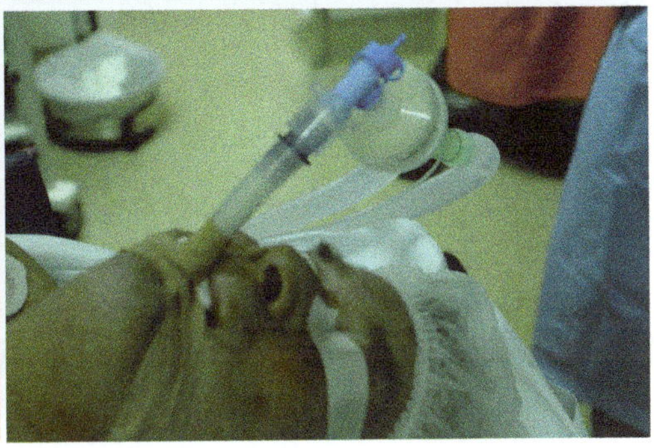

Figure 7.1: Operating theatre setup under local anaesthetic. Author image.

Figure 7.2: Laryngeal mask airway. Author image.

Figure 7.3: Patient under general anaesthetic using LMA. Author image.

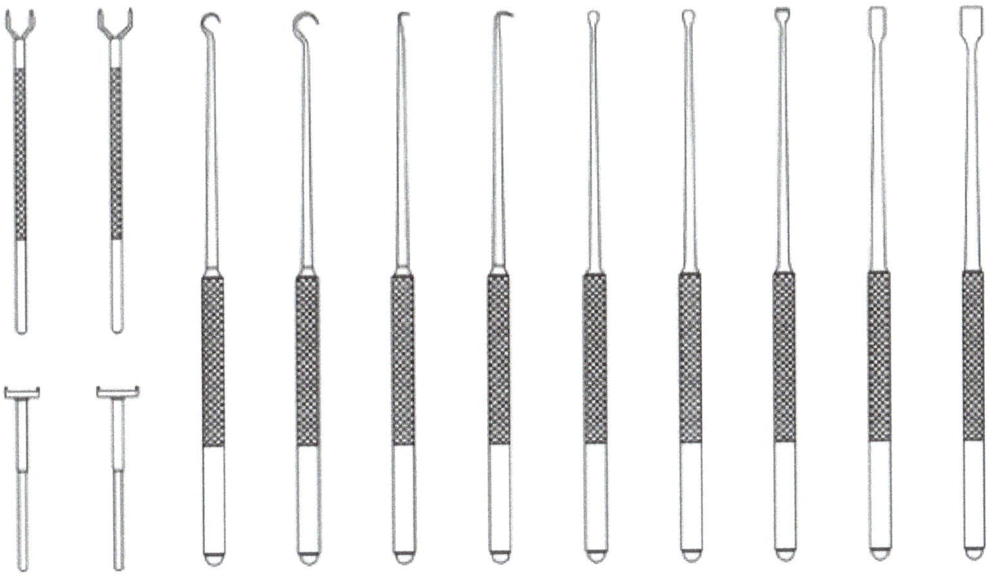

Figure 7.4: Dissecting and measuring tools for MTIS (Kapitex ®Healthcare).

The MTIS comes with either male or female specifically designed sizers for implants, colour coded blue for male and green for female (Figure 7.5). An initial cutting burr (size 4 on average) followed by a smaller (size 2) diamond burr when close to the inner thyroid perichondrium, or a small tangential electrical saw (Stryker® Corp.) can be used to construct the thyroplasty window.

We use quick setting Tissucol fibrin glue (Immuno AG, Baxter®, Deerfield, IL, USA) to cover the window after placement of the stent (Figure 7.6).

Step 4 – Incision and raising of flaps

After the patient is prepared and draped in a sterile setting, a horizontal incision is made, preferably in a neck crease, commencing slightly off midline from the side of surgery close to the inferior margin of the thyroid cartilage (Figure 7.7). Subplatysmal flaps are raised and the deep investing layer of cervical fascia is identified and cut. The strap muscles are retracted laterally and the thyroid cartilage is exposed along the whole lamina with special attention paid to the inferior aspect and visualization of the cricothyroid membrane (Figure 7.8).

Step 5 – Design and construction of window

The landmarks used for the formation of the window are the thyroid notch and the inferior border of the thyroid cartilage. The sizing calliper, depending on the gender of the patient, is used first to locate two points – one anterior and the other posterior to the inferior curve of the thyroid cartilage (Figure 7.9 and Figure 7.10).

A straight line joining these two points is drawn and thereafter the same calliper is placed at the midpoint of the midline of the thyroid cartilage at one end (i.e. between the notch and inferior median border) while the other point of the calliper rests on the line connecting the two aforementioned points. Monopolar diathermy to the calliper and window outline instrument allows for all these landmarks to be seen on the cartilage. This is the 'Key Point' (Figure 7.11).

The window outline instrument is placed such that its antero-superior edge lies on this point and the instrument is laid such that its inferior border is parallel with the inferior edge of the thyroid cartilage. A strut of 2 mm should be preserved between the window and cartilage. Drilling of the window is then performed using a high-speed pneumatic drill with a cutting burr initially (size 4) followed by a smaller diamond burr (size 2) until the inner perichondrium is identified fully but not breached (Figure 7.12).

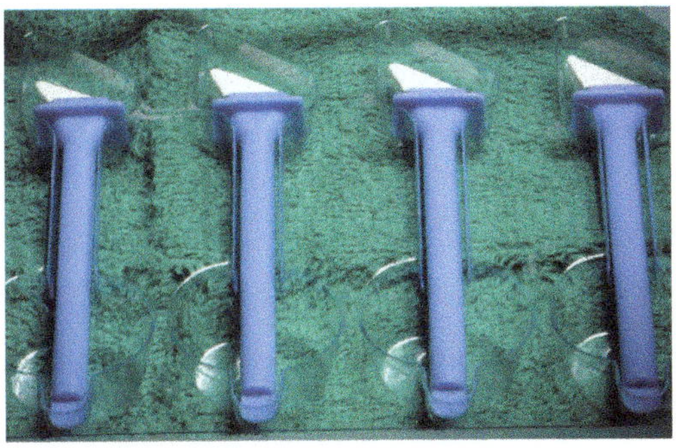

Figure 7.5: Thyroplasty implant sizers for males (Boston®).

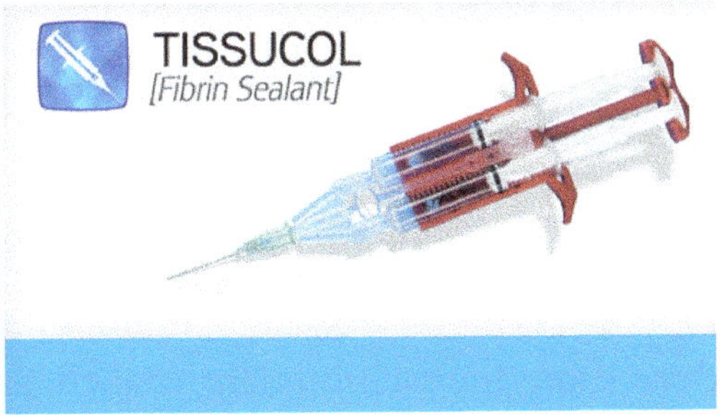

Figure 7.6: Tissucol – Fibrin Sealant. Image courtesy of Baxter®.

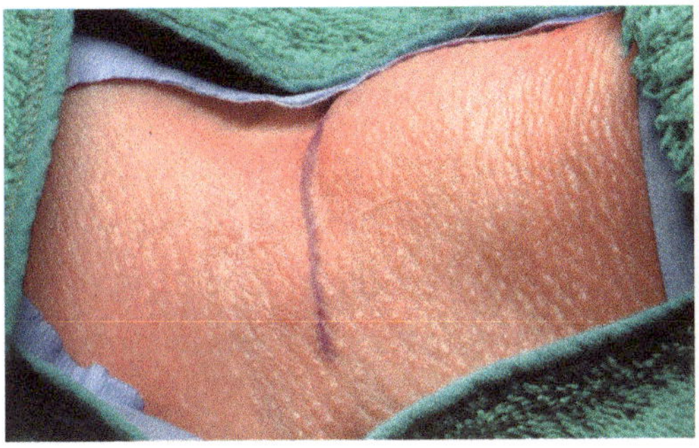

Figure 7.7: Neck prepared with skin marking. Author image.

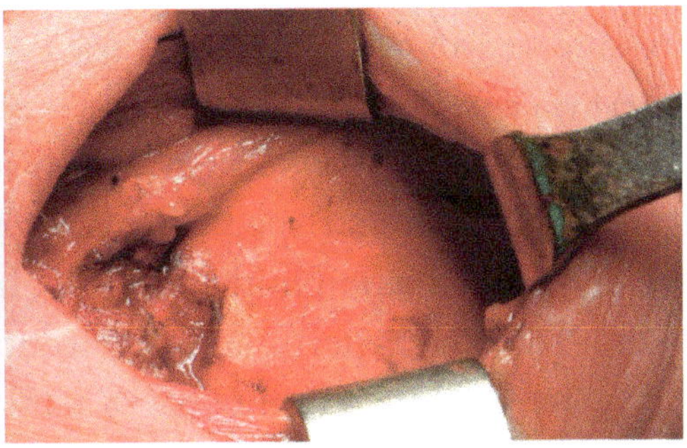

Figure 7.8: Exposure of thyroid cartilage and cricothyroid membrane. Author image.

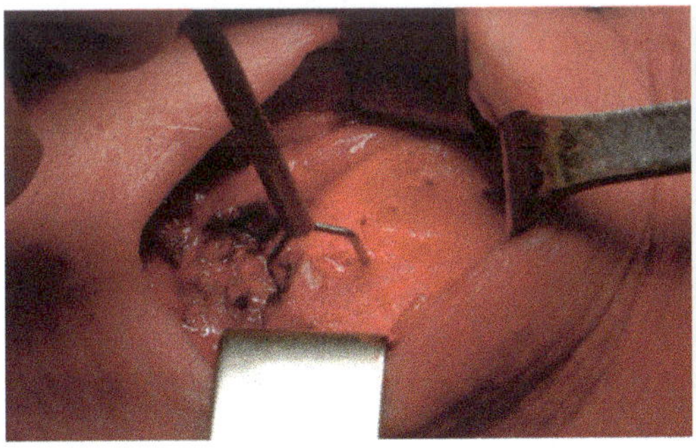

Figure 7.9: First 'mark' made with calliper anterior to inferior curve of thyroid cartilage. Author image.

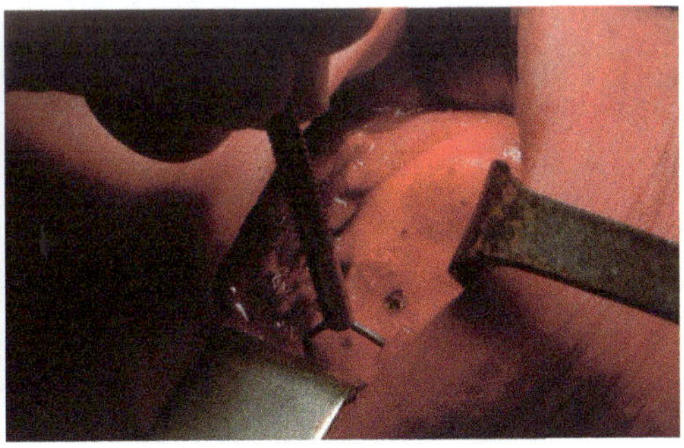

Figure 7.10: Second 'mark' made posterior to inferior thyroid curve. Author image.

Care is taken to release the perichondrium off the thyroid cartilage using the various elevators on the MTIS set. In the case of cordectomies this can prove more fibrotic and difficult.

Step 6 – Measurement of DPSGP and sizing of implant

In cases performed under LA and sedation, the patient is asked to phonate /a/ three times for each implant trialled, at a comfortable pitch and intensity. This enables sizing of the implant, based on both DPSGP and phonation while also under direct visualization of the glottis using a videolaryngoscope. Measurements are recorded by the speech pathologist from an 18 gauge (BD INSYTE-WTM NJ, USA) intravenous cannula in the subglottis connected to an oral pressure sensor of the Phonatory Aerodynamic System (PAS, Kay-Pentax, USA) via a perfusion cable (Figure 7.13 and Figure 7.14).

The implant size is decided by the subjective improvement in voice (by the patient, surgeon, and speech pathologist), the extent of closure of the glottic gap and the reduction in the DPSGP. In GA cases, a flexible videoendoscope is inserted through a port in the connecting tube of the LMA and passed into the larynx to assess the glottic closure achieved using different implant sizes.

Step 7 – Insertion of implant and closure

Once the implant is ready to be inserted, it is grasped with an artery clip and placed posterior, tip first before 'clicking' the anterior aspect with the help of the implant inserter (Figure 7.15 and Figure 7.16). Slow-setting fibrin glue (Tissucol, Immuno AG, Baxter) is then applied around the implant and window site. A small 'mini-vac' suction drain is placed in, prior to closing the wound in two layers. The drain is usually left in situ overnight and removed when there is less than 10 ml collected within.

Post-operative advice and voice therapy

Patients are advised a week of low-intensity voicing after discharge and placed on a 5-day course of broad-spectrum oral antibiotics. All patients undergo voice therapy after surgery to optimize the functional results with the new glottic configuration as described in Chapter 3.

Patients are reviewed in the voice clinic setting a fortnight after the procedure to check on the wound and voice. Thereafter, they are reviewed regularly at six to eight weekly intervals until their voice has been fully optimized.

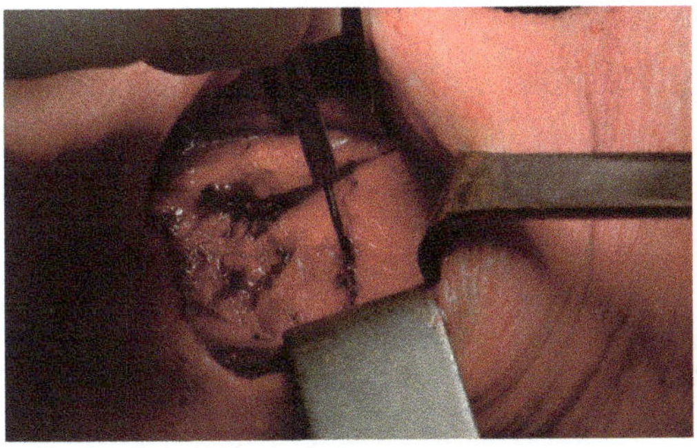

Figure 7.11: 'Key point' located and 'mark' made with monopolar to calliper. Author image.

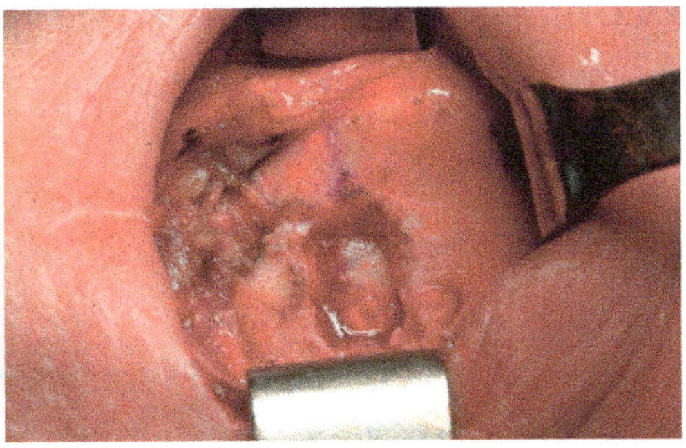

Figure 7.12: Window in thyroid lamina drilled. Author image.

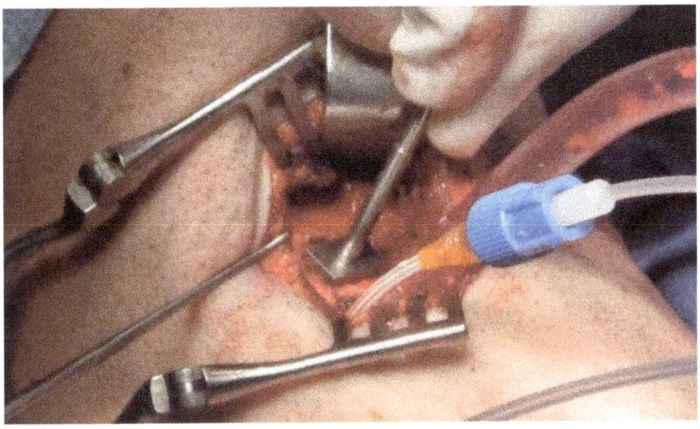

Figure 7.13: Trans-cricothyroid cannula with window implement above. Author image.

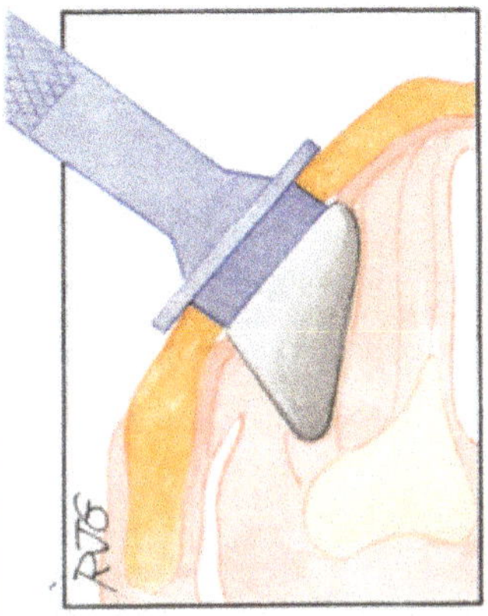

Figure 7.14: Schematic diagram of sizer in thyroplasty window. Image courtesy of Boston Medical Products.

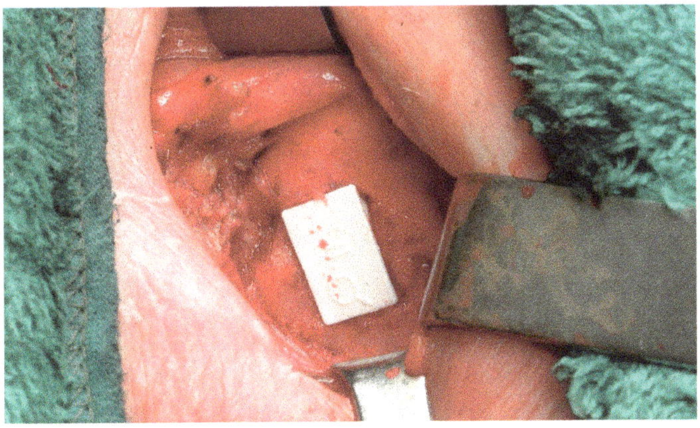

Figure 7.15: Implant in window. Author image.

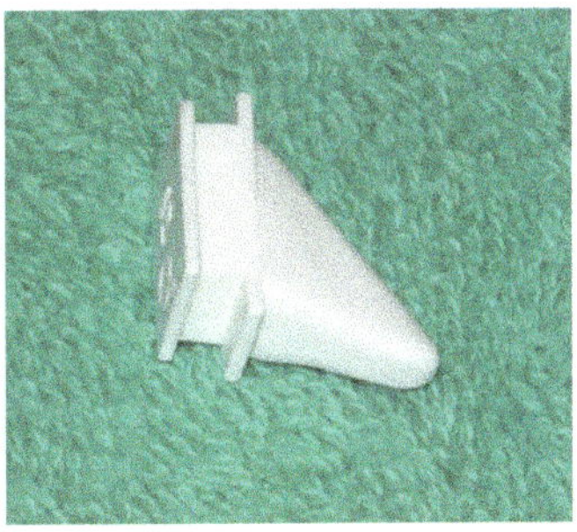

Figure 7.16: Implant prior to insertion. Author image..

Common pitfalls and mistakes

- Incision made too high and not fully exposing the inferior border of the thyroid.
- Window not parallel to the inferior border of thyroid.
- No strut, or insufficient strut, between window and inferior border of thyroid.
- Dissection of perichondrium breaching neocord or soft tissue.
- Window made too high or implant inserted at an angle, medializing the ventricular fold.

Tips and pearls

- Type I thyroplasty using the Montgomery system should be considered for narrowing both the anterior and posterior glottic gap.
- The thyroid cartilage lamina should be exposed fully with a good view of the inferior border and cricothyroid membrane.
- Excessive dissection within the window and breach of the inner perichondrium or neocord can increase glottic oedema which may falsely improve voice improvement.

Further reading

Cummings C, Purcell L, Flint P. 1993. Hydroxylapatite laryngeal implants for medialization. Preliminary report. *Ann Otol Rhinol Laryngol* **102**:843–51.

Friedrich G. 1999. Titanium vocal fold medializing implant – introducing a novel implant system for external vocal fold medialization. *Ann Otol Rhinol Laryngol* **108**:79–86.

Friedrich G, de Jong FI, Mahieu HF, et al. 2001. Laryngeal framework surgery: a proposal for classification and nomenclature by the Phonosurgery Committee of the European Laryngological Society. *Eur Arch Otorhinolaryngol* **258**:389–96.

Giovanni A, Demolin D, Heim C, et al. 2000. Estimated subglottic pressure in normal and dysphonic subjects. *Ann Otol Rhinol Laryngol* **109**(5):500–4.

Isshiki N, Morita H, Okamura H, et al. 1974. Thyroplasty as a new phonosurgical technique. *Acta Otolaryngol* **78**:451–7.

Isshiki N. 1989. *Phonosurgery: Theory and Practice.* Tokyo: Springer.

Ketelslagers K, De Bodt MS, Wuyts FL, et al. 2007. Relevance of subglottic pressure in normal and dysphonic subjects. *Eur Arch Otorhinolaryngol* **264**(5):519–23.

Mastronikolis NS, Remacle M, Kiagiadaki D et al. 2013. Medialization thyroplasty for voice restoration after transoral cordectomy. *Eur Arch Otorhinolaryngol* **270**:2071–8.

Matar N, Remacle M, Bachy V et al. 2012. Objective measurement of real time subglottic pressure during medialization thyroplasty: a feasibility study. *Eur Arch Otorhinolaryngol* **269**(4):1171–5.

Montgomery WW, Blaugrund SM, Varvares MA. 1993. Thyroplasty: a new approach. *Ann Otol Rhinol Laryngol* **102**:571–9.

Montgomery WW, Montgomery SK. 1997. Montgomery Thyroplasty Implant System. *Ann Otol Rhinol Laryngol* (Suppl) **106**:170.

Remacle M, Lawson G, Hedayat A, et al. 2001. Medialization framework surgery for voice improvement after endoscopic cordectomy. *Eur Arch Otorhinolaryngol* **258**:267–71.

Remacle M, Lawson G, Morsomme D, et al. 2006. Reconstruction of glottic defects after endoscopic cordectomy: voice outcome. *Otolaryngol Clin North Am* **39**:191–204.

Remacle M, Eckel HE, Antonelli A, et al. 2000. Endoscopic cordectomy. A proposal for a classification by the Working Committee European Laryngological Society. *Eur Arch Otorhinolaryngol* **257**:227–31.

8

Arytenoid adduction

Nupur Kapoor Nerurkar and Jayakumar Menon

Indications

Unilateral vocal fold palsy with breathy dysphonia, which is not amenable to treatment by type I thyroplasty alone, is the indication for arytenoid adduction (AA) also referred to as arytenoid rotation (AR) (Figure 8.1). Usually, unilateral vocal fold palsy is corrected by medialization thyroplasty. However, when there is big posterior phonatory gap, especially with a vertical level incompatibility, the malrotated arytenoid often needs to be corrected with an arytenoid adduction procedure. As of now, there are no definite ways to predict the need of the arytenoid adduction pre-operatively. The final decision is always taken on the operation table.

Contraindications

Cricoarytenoid joint dislocation is a contraindication for AA.

An irradiated larynx is a relative contraindication as the radiation-induced fibrosis may increase the risk of pyriform mucosa tear during dissection.

Occasionally, a patient may develop stridor during the AA procedure and this may then have to be abandoned.

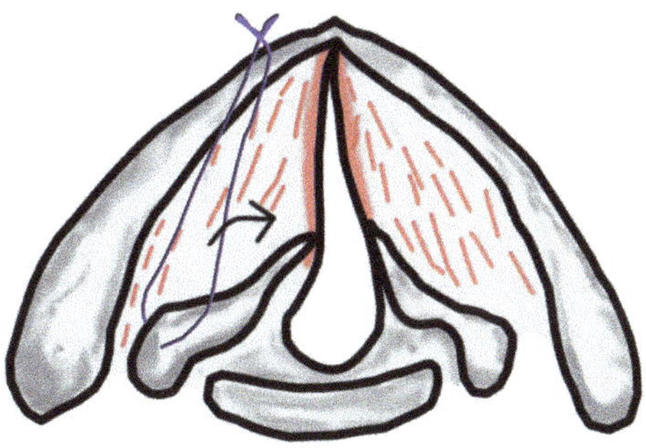

Figure 8.1: Principle for arytenoid adduction. Author image.

Clinical anatomy

The cricoarytenoid joint is a saddle type of synovial joint. Two types of movements are possible. First is a gliding type of movement supero-medially (adduction) and infero-laterally (abduction). This is essentially controlled by the interarytenoid muscles which have a bilateral innervation. It is exceedingly rare to have total denervation of this muscle and, hence, this movement is not commonly affected. The second movement is more complicated and is a sort of rotatory movement of the body of the arytenoid on the cricoid around a vertical axis. This action brings the tip of the vocal process to and away from the vocal process of the opposite side. It is easy to understand that the type I thyroplasty cannot bring about this effect.

Physiology

The arytenoid cartilages are acted upon by three groups of muscles. The first group comprises the muscles supplied by the ipsilateral recurrent laryngeal nerve. These are the posterior cricoarytenoid, lateral cricoarytenoid, and thyroarytenoid. The second group contains the interarytenoid which has innervations from both ipsi and contralateral recurrent laryngeal nerves. Cricothyroid, supplied by the superior laryngeal nerve, is the third group. So it is obvious that in case of unilateral recurrent laryngeal nerve palsy the arytenoid is subjected to an unopposed pull of interarytenoid and cricothyroid muscles. In addition, depending upon the severity of the nerve injury and regeneration as well as synkinesis, even the muscles in the first group can act upon the arytenoid in different ways. This is why each unilateral vocal fold palsy produces different arytenoid positions, and why each has to be addressed differently. An arytenoid, which assumed a particular position immediately after the nerve injury, may shift to a different position later on, precisely due to the same reason.

History

Nobuhiko Isshiki described his approach to the arytenoid and dislocated the cricothyroid joint and, if needed, removed a rim of posterior thyroid ala. He also advocated partial opening of the cricoarytenoid joint.

Nowadays, it is uncommon to open the cricoarytenoid joint for arytenoid adduction; however, it is resorted to for adduction arytenoidopexy. Nick Maragos described a way to avoid the cricothyroid joint dislocation by cutting a window on the posterior thyroid ala. This, he suggested, was more physiological.

Pre-operative work up

A thorough history is taken with special emphasis on onset of dysphonia, possible etiological factors, and its impact on patient's communication ability. See Chapter 3 for assessment details. Voice Handicap Index is determined and the patient's voice is perceptually analysed as well as recorded. Maximum phonation time (MPT) is noted; however, computerized voice analysis is optional and not always performed by the authors.

Flexible laryngoscopy is performed to assess the relative or absolute immobility of the vocal fold. The position of the arytenoids during phonation is ascertained. The phonatory gap and bowing of the vocal fold, if any, are also noted. An attempt is made to ascertain vertical level incompatibility, as the paralysed vocal fold is likely to be at a higher level in many cases. It is also very important to make sure that the opposite vocal fold is abducting well, as the absence of this will result in stridor when AA is performed.

Stroboscopic evaluation using a rigid scope will give valuable clues regarding the integrity of the Reinke's space. If the Reinke's space is scarred, even a perfect arytenoid adduction and medialization thyroplasty may not give good results.

A CT scan is performed to rule out any pathology along the route of the recurrent laryngeal nerve in apparently idiopathic cases. Very rarely, if there is a suspicion of arytenoid dislocation, either a laryngeal EMG or palpation of the cricoarytenoid joints under general anaesthesia may be required.

Consent

The pathology and the plan of surgery must be explained to the patient. Sharing the laryngoscopy video will be helpful for this purpose. The patient needs to be informed of the possibility of suboptimal outcomes, the possibility of requiring further surgery, and the abandonment of the AA procedure if respiratory distress develops. The patient should also be made aware of the value of postoperative voice therapy.

If the pyriform fossa mucosa is breached, the patient will have to be on a feeding tube for a week or so. Though this is very uncommon, the patient should be informed about this, as well as the possibility of transient breathing difficulty secondary to oedema or haematoma.

The patient should also be instructed not to undergo any elective endotracheal intubation or upper gastrointestinal endoscopy for at least six weeks post-operatively, or risk disrupting the arytenoid adduction effect. If an emergency intubation is needed, a smaller endotracheal tube is advocated.

Operative procedure

Step 1 – Anaesthetic technique

Arytenoid adduction is often performed along with a type I thyroplasty. Both these procedures require the operating surgeon to talk to and hear the voice of the patient in response to the medialization, in order to ascertain the optimum medialization needed for the patient. It is thus of paramount importance that the patient be operated under local anaesthesia with mild sedation. That is, enough sedation to allay the surgical anxiety, but not such that the patient starts snoring or mumbling incoherently. See also Chapter 5.

Step 2 – Position

The patient is supine and is given a head and neck extension in order to make the laryngeal cartilages more prominent and palpable. A slight head elevation and a pillow under the knees may make the patient more comfortable.

Step 3 – Specific equipment

Besides a basic surgical tray needed for open neck surgery, the specific instruments needed for AA are a piriform mucosa elevator, mastoid suction with adaptor, blunt single cricoid hook, ethmoid/sphenoid/Kerrison's punch, turbinectomy scissors, and 4-0 prolene suture on a round body needle. A bipolar and unipolar cautery should also be available. Neurosurgical patties dipped in 4% lidocaine with adrenaline are helpful during elevation of the piriform mucosa. Figure 8.3 shows the specific instruments one should keep ready prior to the procedure. A flexible laryngoscope and 4% lidocaine spray are also required during this procedure.

Step 4 – Incision

As most arytenoid adduction procedures complement a type I thyroplasty, the skin incision has already been made, preferably in a prominent skin crease over the thyroid cartilage and laterally extending to the lateral border of the thyroid

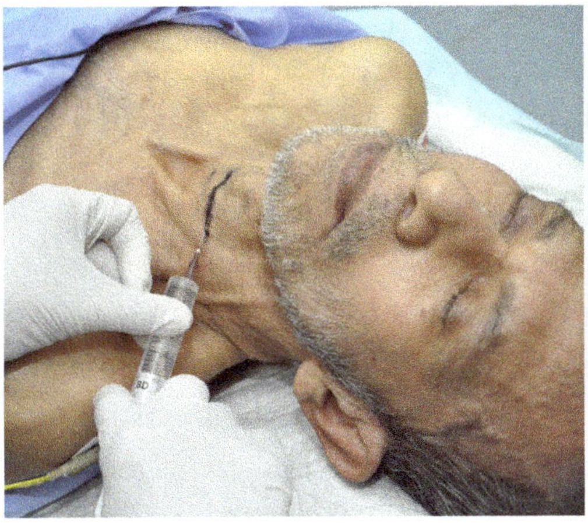

Figure 8.2: Positioning and infiltration. Image courtesy Nerurkar, Menon.

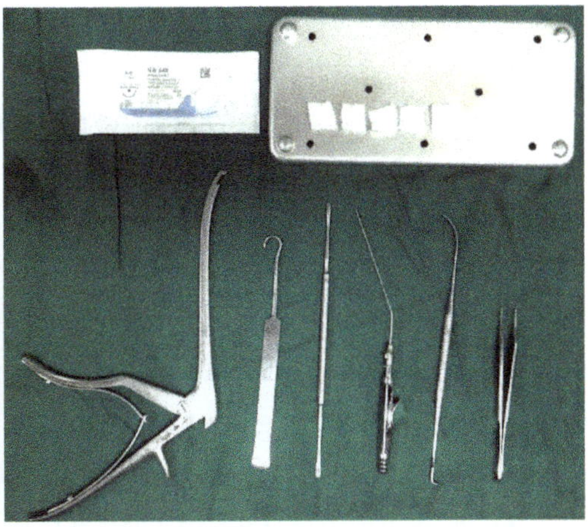

Figure 8.3: Specific instruments needed for AA. Image courtesy Nerurkar, Menon.

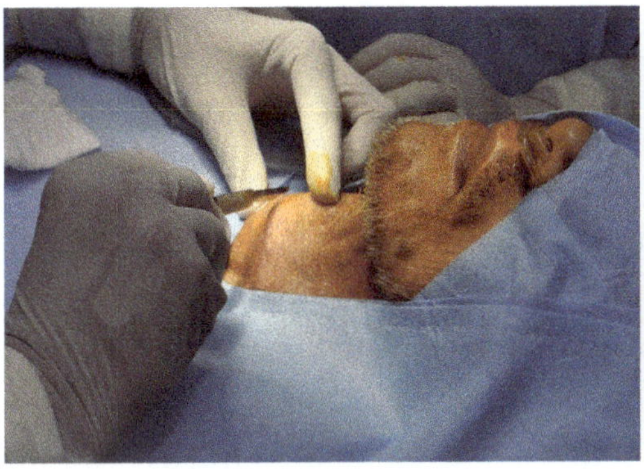

Figure 8.4: Incision. Image courtesy Nerurkar, Menon.

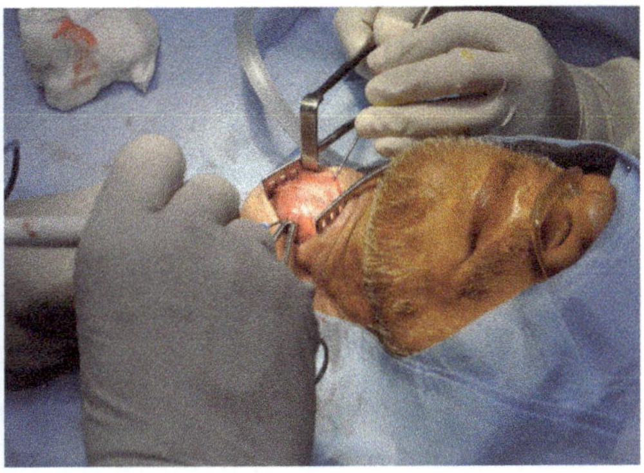

Figure 8.5: Dividing strap muscles. Image courtesy Nerurkar, Menon.

cartilage (Figure 8.4). Following subplatysmal flap elevation, the thyroid ala of the side being operated on is exposed completely. The strap muscles are often not divided for a type I thyroplasty. Once the decision to perform an arytenoid adduction is taken, the strap muscles are divided between two haemostatic clamps and the raw edges cauterized (Figure 8.5). A window in the thyroid cartilage has already been created for a type I thyroplasty and medialization through this window does not produce any/satisfactory voice improvement and posterior phonatory gap closure. This is when one proceeds to perform the arytenoid adduction procedure.

Step 5 – Dissection to expose the arytenoid.

Approaches for arytenoid adduction/rotation are open procedures that may or may not involve dislocation of the cricothyroid and cricoarytenoid joint. Arytenopexy procedure, however, does warrant cricoarytenoid joint dissection.

In the author's view, the simplest and most easily reproducible approach to the arytenoid is via the creation of the Maragos window. This approach does not require opening of the cricothyroid or cricoarytenoid joints.

A C-shaped incision is made to cut the outer perichondrium of the thyroid cartilage with a cutting cautery from the base of the superior cornu to the base of the inferior cornu going beyond the oblique line of the thyroid cartilage (Figure 8.6). A perichondrial elevator is used to elevate this outer perichondrium along with all the muscles attached to the oblique line, from the thyroid ala up to the lateral edge of the cartilage, with minimal bleeding (Figure 8.7).

The cautery is now used to separate the lateral edge of the thyroid cartilage from the constrictor muscles. This is done from around 1 cm below the superior cornu attachment for a variable length of 23 cm (depending on the size of the cartilage).

A blunt single cricoid hook is used to retract medially the lateral edge of the thyroid cartilage of the side being operated on. The piriform fossa mucosa is now gradually separated from the thyroid inner perichondrium from this lateral edge of the thyroid cartilage using a piriform fossa elevator and neurosurgical patties soaked in 4% lidocaine with adrenaline. As the piriform mucosa is elevated (in a cranial and posterior direction), a C-shaped Maragos window is created by removing the thyroid cartilage that has been separated from the piriform mucosa (Figure 8.8). The size of this window is variable depending on the size of the thyroid ala, however a height and width of 3–3.5 cm is adequate. Care should be taken to maintain a minimum of 5 cm between the Maragos window and the thyroplasty window so that the intervening cartilage does not fracture during dissection or implant placement (Figure 8.9).

The muscular process of the arytenoid is now palpated (Figure 8.10), in the dissection bed, as the arytenoid is better felt than seen at this stage. It feels to the palpating finger as a raw rice grain. Dissection with a fine haemostat is performed over this area of the muscular process by holding the muscular attachments to the muscular process of the arytenoid and not the cartilage itself, which has a tendency to break. The shiny white cartilage of the muscular process slowly reveals itself. At this stage it is important to confirm that this is not the

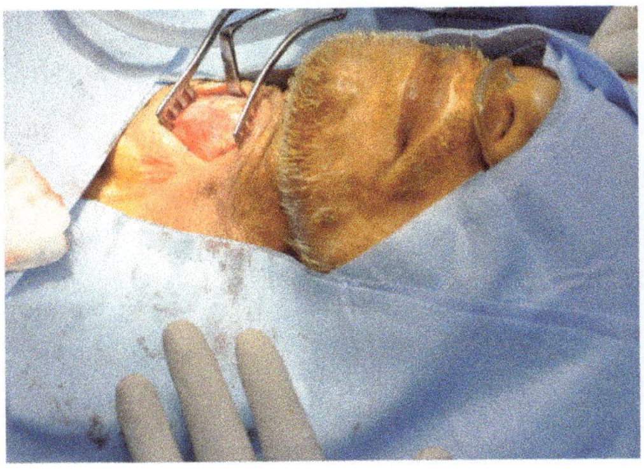

Figure 8.6: Flap raised. Image courtesy Nerurkar, Menon.

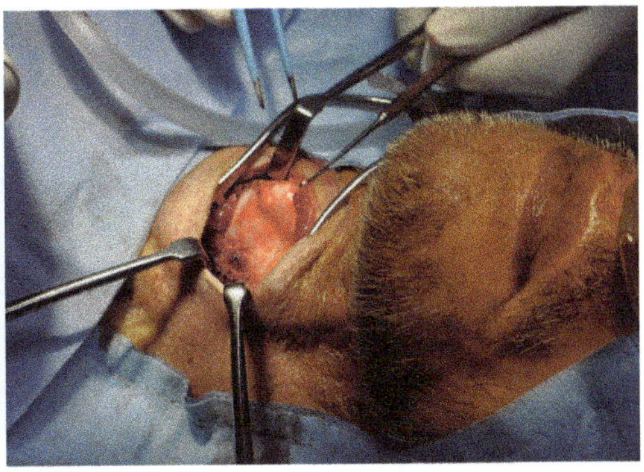

Figure 8.7: Skeletonizing the larynx. Image courtesy Nerurkar, Menon.

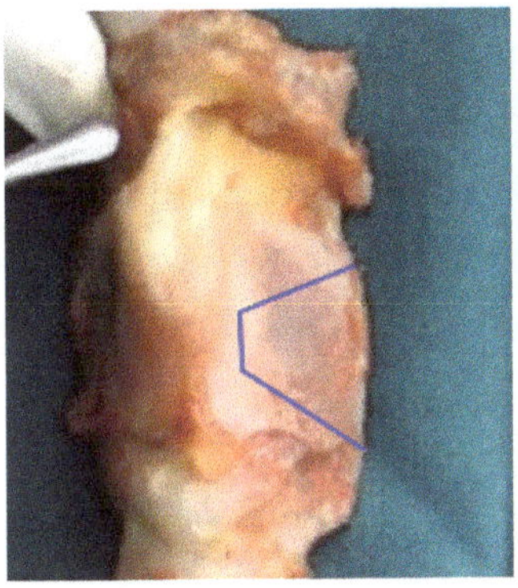

Figure 8.8: C-shaped window (Maragos window). Image courtesy Nerurkar, Menon.

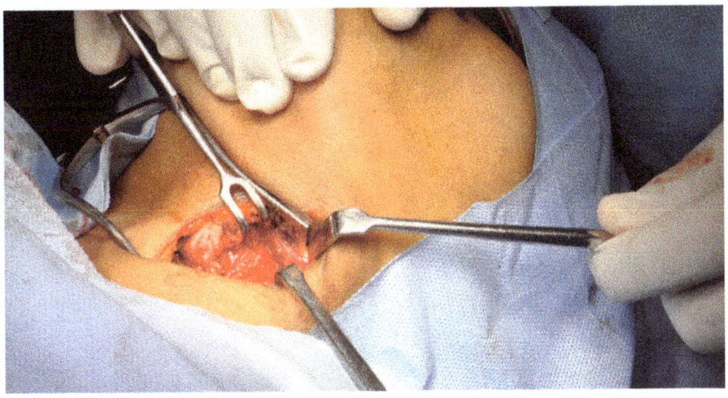

Figure 8.9: Maragos window completed. Image courtesy Nerurkar, Menon.

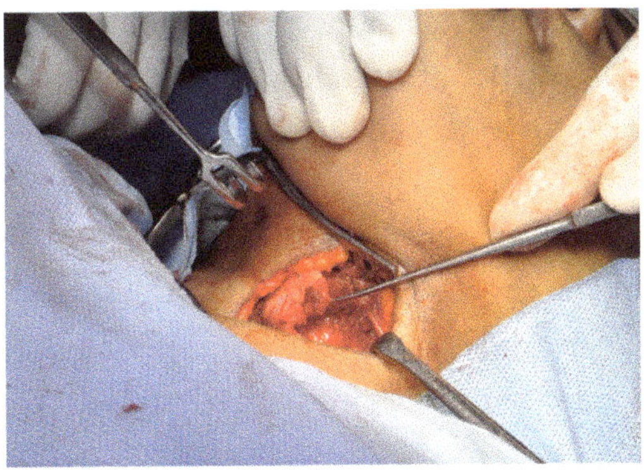

Figure 8.10: Palpating for the muscular process of the arytenoids. Image courtesy Nerurkar, Menon.

cricoid cartilage. A flexible laryngoscope is introduced after spraying the nostrils with 4% lidocaine. The muscular attachments of the arytenoid are held with a plain forceps and gently moved, thus moving the arytenoid. This movement of the arytenoid is confirmed on flexible laryngoscopy.

Step 6 – Arytenoid adduction suture placement

A 3-O or a 4-O prolene suture is used to take a 'figure of 8' stitch through the muscular process of the arytenoid cartilage. Holding the lateral cricoarytenoid muscle with a plain forceps, the needle of the prolene suture is passed into the muscular process twice (creating a figure of 8) and a knot may be tied at this time (Figure 8.11).

Now both the needle and non-needle threads of this prolene suture are fed into the thyroplasty window from underneath the cartilage strut separating the Maragos window from the thyroplasty window (Figure 8.12).

The needle end is now passed from the thyroplasty window through the midline of the thyroid cartilages as near to the cricothyroid membrane as possible (Figure 8.12) and the non-needle thread is now passed under the 3 mm lower rim of cartilage.

Step 7 – Tying the knot

Both the ends of the thread are now pulled anteroinferiorly and the patient is asked to phonate. Depending on when the patient's voice appears the strongest the knot is tied. This is usually a loose knot (the tip of the haemostat can pass below it, which tightens, on phonation) (Figure 8.13).

When arytenoid adduction is being performed with a type I thyroplasty, the implant is placed after the arytenoid adduction stitch has been made and this implant lies over the two threads passing through the thyroplasty window (Figure 8.14).

In addition to hearing a strong voice of the patient at the conclusion of the surgery, a final flexible laryngoscopic view should confirm good closure of the phonatory gap with arytenoid symmetry during phonation. There should be no vertical level mismatch between the two vocal folds.

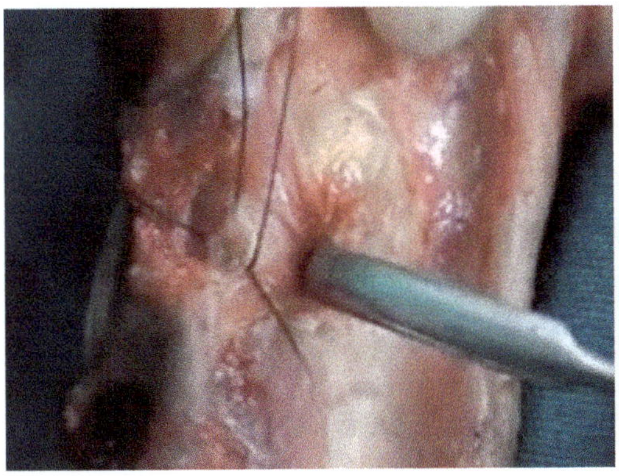

Figure 8.11: 'Figure of 8' suture being taken through the left muscular process in a cadaver dissection. Image courtesy Nerurkar, Menon.

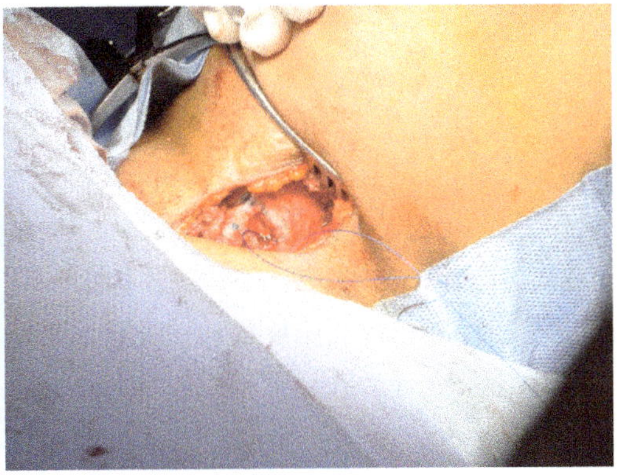

Figure 8.12: Needle and non-needle threads of prolene suture that have been fed into the thyroplasty window. Image courtesy Nerurkar, Menon.

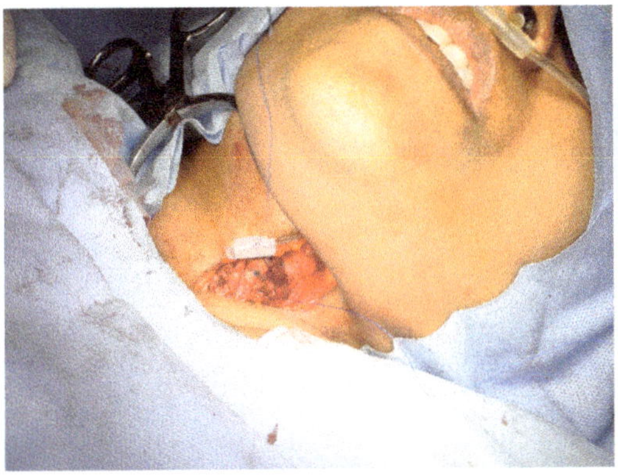

Figure 8.13: Arytenoid sutures passed through type I implant. Image courtesy Nerurkar, Menon.

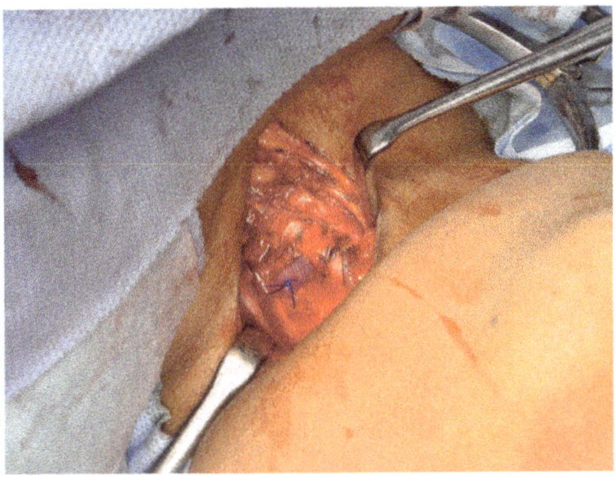

Figure 8.14: Final position of implant with suture. Image courtesy Nerurkar, Menon.

Step 8 – Closure

Before closure, a drain is placed at the operative site and any piriform mucosa tear is looked for by placing 5–10 ml of saline over the piriform mucosa and asking the patient to blow (as if blowing birthday candles) to balloon up the piriform mucosa.

In case of a piriform mucosa tear, bubbles will be seen. The mucosa should be repaired by suturing it and a nasogastric tube inserted.

The strap muscles are now re-sutured and two-layer closure is performed. A dressing may be placed if required, after antibiotic ointment is applied to the incision site.

Post-operative management

The authors give a broad-spectrum antibiotic intravenously during the procedure and for 48 hours post-operatively. The patient is put on oral antibiotics after 48 hours, for one week. Intravenous steroids are given intra-operatively and occasionally post-operatively if the arytenoid oedema is extensive. Anti-inflammatory medication and anti-reflux medication for one week is recommended to all patients. If the patient displays any difficulty in swallowing saliva, or any doubt regarding piriform mucosa integrity, a fibreoptic endoscopic evaluation of swallowing (FEES) is performed prior to giving oral feeds. Routinely, the authors start oral feeds six hours after surgery. The patient is typically discharged 48 hours after the procedure, once the drain is serous in nature. The first post-operative visit is at seven days, when the single continuous subcuticular suture is removed and a laryngoscopy performed.

The patient is advised post-operative voice rest for 48 hours followed by limited vocal use in a confidential voice for a week. A few sessions of voice therapy are suggested three to four weeks after the procedure.

Complications and pitfalls

- Tearing the piriform mucosa is a real possibility. By asking the patient to blow during dissection, the integrity of this mucosa can be confirmed. If a patty is placed over the mucosa pushing it superiorly and posteriorly, trauma can be avoided. In case of a tear, the mucosa must be sutured and a feeding tube put in. The patient is not given oral feeds until FEES confirms good passage of liquids and solids.
- Fracturing the rim of cartilage between the thyroplasty window and the Maragos window may take place, especially if it is less than 1 cm in width. Repairing this can be challenging but must be attempted so that the implant is not destabilized. The authors recommend suturing a knot on either side of the fracture and then tying these two threads to one another.
- Fracturing the muscular process of the arytenoid may occur if held directly. Holding the LCA muscle avoids fracturing the muscular process of the arytenoid.
- Bleeding during the procedure must be controlled locally and by the anaesthetist as the chances of piriform mucosa tear and other complications will increase.

- Occasionally, the arytenoid adduction stitch may cause respiratory distress and stridor in the patient and must then be abandoned. Intravenous steroids are recommended at the time of dissection itself. The authors have not had a case that needed to be abandoned due to stridor, but two female patients complained of snoring post-procedure. A sleep study did not suggest a significant sleep apnoea in either patient.
- Mistaking the cricoid as the arytenoid is avoided by a flexible laryngoscopic check.
- A very tight AA stitch will cause a strained voice and must be avoided. The AA sutures must also not get caught on any uneven or sharp points in the Maragos or thyroplasty window, as this will change the vector forces of the AA stitch.

Tips and pearls

- Arytenoid adduction is an on-table decision to be taken when a type I thyroplasty does not improve the patient's voice.
- It is more likely to be performed in patients who have a MPT of less than five seconds, a large posterior phonatory gap, a level mismatch of the vocal folds, arytenoid asymmetry on phonation, and in revision thyroplasty cases.
- In the authors' experience, 30% of type I thyroplasty procedures also need an arytenoid adduction procedure.
- The learning curve for arytenoid adduction procedures is longer than that for type I thyroplasty, and cadaver dissections and observing live surgery is strongly recommended.
- Creation of an adequately large Maragos window allows for a comfortable AA stitch placement.

Further reading

Ishhikki N, Tanabe M, Sawada M. 1998. Arytenoid adduction for unilateral vocal cord paralysis. *Arch Otolaryngol* **104**(10):555.

Maragos NE. 1999. The posterior thyroplasty window: anatomical considerations. *Laryngoscope* **109**(8): 1228–31.

Slavit DH, Maragos NE. 1992. Physiologic assessment of arytenoid adduction. *Ann Otol Rhino Laryngol* **101**:321–7.

Weinman EC, Maragos NE. 2000. Airway compromise in thyroplasty surgery. *Laryngoscope* **110**(7):1082–1085.

Zeitels SM, Hochman I, Hillman RE. 1998. Adduction arytenopexy: a new procedure for paralytic dysphonia with implications for implant medialisation. *Ann Otol Rhinol Laryngol* **173**:2–24.

9

Injection medialization laryngoplasty

Mark Watson and Jane Shaw

Introduction

Injection laryngoplasty (IL) is one of the treatment options for glottic insufficiency. Over the last decade, it has become an increasingly popular alternative to type I thyroplasty, as outcomes have been shown to be similar in many patients. Conditions producing glottic insufficiency include:

- unilateral vocal cord palsy;
- vocal cord paresis (including the possible need for 'top up' after previous intervention);
- presbyphonia/vocal cord atrophy;
- vocal cord defects following previous treatment (e.g. cordectomy or radiotherapy for early tumours); and
- vocal cord scar or sulcus.

Patient assessment

Patients presenting with dysphonia due to glottic insufficiency should undergo a full voice clinic assessment from a laryngologist and speech therapist. The duration and severity of symptoms are important, as well as the presence of other underlying disease (e.g. vocal cord palsy due to lung cancer). The occupation and vocal demand of each patient are crucial when deciding on management options. Examination should include videostroboscopy with either a rigid or flexible digital laryngoscope with video recording. The size of the glottic gap should be noted, along with the cord position in cord palsy cases.

Most specialists would document each case before and after treatment using a combination of a patient-reported symptom scale (e.g. VHI, VHI-10, VoiSS) and a perceptual analysis of voice (e.g. GRBAS, CAPE-V). In terms of acoustic parameters, perhaps maximum phonation time is of greatest relevance to glottic insufficiency.

Treatment options

Not all patients with glottic insufficiency require operative intervention. An elderly patient with presbyphonia and little vocal demand, for instance, may simply require assurance that their dysphonia is not related to any sinister underlying disease process. Many patients may benefit from voice therapy in the first instance, with operative intervention being reserved for those who do not respond adequately. In other cases, the large time investment in, and duration of, a course of voice therapy may be unacceptable. This may either be because of expected limited survival in a patient with lung cancer, or due to occupational or social factors, and the relatively 'quick fix' provided by IL may be preferable.

When IL is indicated, further options need to be considered. Should the procedure be carried out under local or general anaesthesia? Which material should be injected, to produce a shorter or longer duration of action? For LA techniques, which approach should be used?

Choice of anaesthesia

There has been a fairly rapid trend over the last decade for an increasing number of IL procedures to be performed under local anaesthesia (LA) on an awake patient, often in an ambulatory setting ('in-office') rather than the more traditional approach involving microlaryngoscopy under general anaesthesia (GA).

Local anaesthesia has the advantage of avoiding the complications, cost and inconvenience of GA, and can allow procedures to be performed in subjects who are not fit for GA. On the other hand, GA may be more suitable in some cases due to patient tolerance, anatomical factors such as neck scarring after previous treatment or an overhanging arytenoid, or functional issues such as false cord hyperfunction, which would make access for an LA technique difficult. Some materials require high-pressure injection via a broad-gauge needle, which means that GA is required and, when fat is used, GA is needed to allow harvest (usually from the abdomen).

Patients should be warned that there is always a small risk of airway compromise during an injection. In theory, this should be very small as IL can only medialize the membranous part of the cord, anterior to the vocal process of the arytenoid, leaving the posterior third of the glottis (which is the most important part of the laryngeal airway) largely unaffected. LA procedures involve incremental injection of small aliquots of material until the desired result is obtained and so, in theory, should be even less risky in this respect.

If IL is to be performed outside of an operating theatre, it is important that the setting chosen reaches an adequate safety standard in terms of proximity to other hospital services, staffing, equipment, monitoring, and back-up services in case of problems. In the UK, standards for in-office laryngeal procedures have been set by ENT-UK.

Although serious complications of IL are rare, caution must be exercised in patients taking anticoagulant drugs. Generally, such drugs should be stopped, if possible, several days prior to IL.

Choice of injection material

The first description of IL was by Brünings in 1911, using paraffin wax. In the 1970s and 1980s, Teflon paste was used, but was found to cause granuloma formation in many patients and is no longer in use. The range of injection material currently available for IL includes:

Short term

- gelfoam
- carboxymethylcellulose
- collagen (bovine or human)
- hyaluronic acid
- autologous fat.

Long term

- calcium hydroxylapatite
- Bioplastique
- autologous fat.

It will be noted that fat has been included as a both a short- or a long-term option due to its variable survival. Most of the short-term materials last for between two and six months, as opposed to much longer periods for the long-term products.

One of the great advantages of short-term injections is that they can be used early in the course of vocal cord palsy, when there is still a good chance that cord movement may recover. They can also be used as a 'test drive' so that a patient can experience the benefits of vocal cord medialization before deciding whether they wish to undergo long-term medialization, either by IL or open surgery. Interestingly, it has been shown that early IL with a short-term material significantly reduces the need for long-term medialization even when cord mobility never recovers.

Choice of approach

For LA procedures, the injection can be delivered via a transoral, transendoscopic or percutaneous route. Transoral injections are popular with some authors, particularly when rigid laryngoscopy is used. A curved needle is passed alongside the laryngoscope and directed toward the upper surface of the cord. Transendoscopic procedures via a flexible endoscope rely on finding an endoscopic injection needle which is sufficiently rigid to pierce the laryngeal mucosa to the necessary depth while being of sufficiently wide bore to reduce resistance to injection: to date, the author has not yet found the ideal needle.

UK practice at present uses mainly percutaneous techniques. Under digital flexible endoscopic control, the injection may be placed via the cricothyroid membrane, the thyrohyoid membrane, or directly through the thyroid cartilage ala (Figure 9.1).

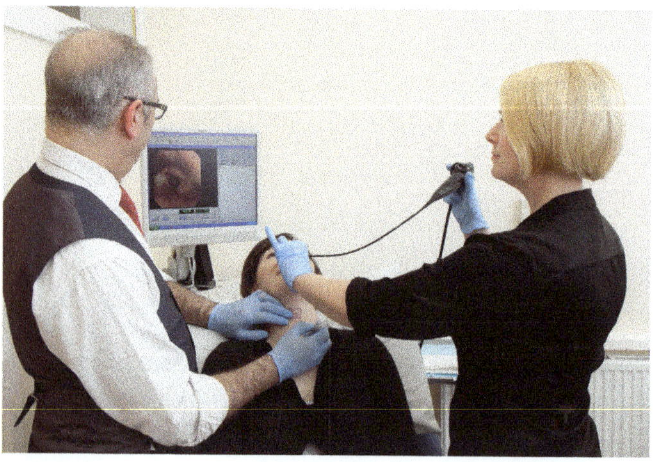

Figure 9.1: Injection set up in the outpatient department. Image courtesy Watson and Shaw.

The transcricothyroid technique (Figure 9.2) approaches the vocal cord from below, whereas the transthyrohyoid technique (Figure 9.3) approaches from above. The transthyroid cartilage approach (Figure 9.4) reaches the thyroarytenoid muscle directly without the needle entering the lumen.

All of the percutaneous techniques are a little more difficult in female rather than male subjects as the cricoid and thyroid cartilages are more difficult to palpate, especially in obese individuals. The transcricothyroid technique can be more difficult if the larynx is lying low in the neck, or there is significant kyphosis or stiff neck, as some extension is helpful. The transthyrohyoid approach can be difficult if there is a large chin, and sometimes the needle enters the lumen parallel to the surface of the cords, so actually penetrating the cord in order to inject can be difficult. The transthyroid cartilage approach can be limited by ossification in the cartilage itself. Although each laryngeal surgeon will develop their 'favourite' approach, it is important to be trained in all approaches, as each individual case may require a tailor-made treatment.

With all variations of technique it is vital that the injected material is delivered into the thyroarytenoid muscle lateral to the vocal ligament. Injection into Reinke's space will destroy the mucosal wave and produce a very poor voice, which may require cordotomy to remove some of the longer-lasting agents.

Procedure techniques

General anaesthesia

A standard suspension microlaryngoscopy is performed. GA may be supported by endotracheal intubation, or a tubeless method using jet ventilation. The vocal

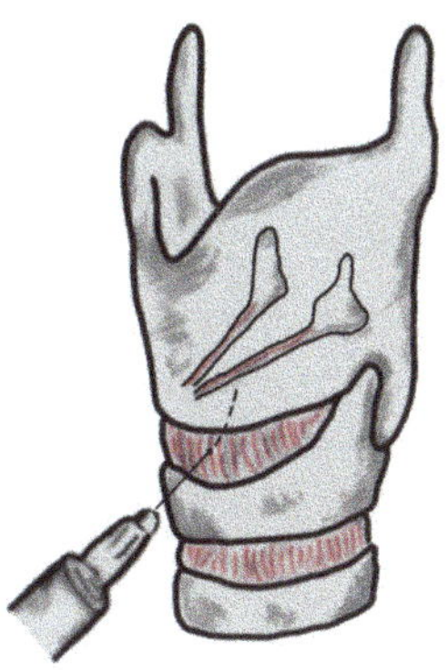

Figure 9.2: Transcricothyroid approach. Author image.

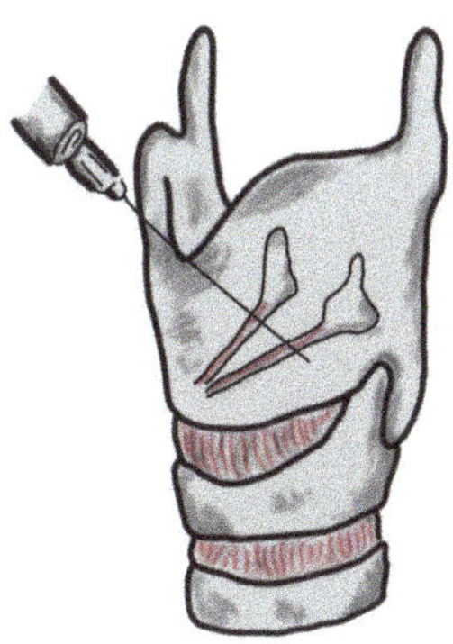

Figure 9.3: Transthyrohyoid approach. Author image.

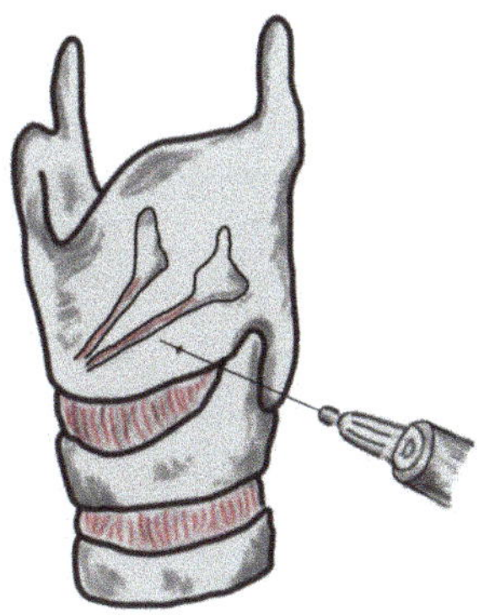

Figure 9.4: Transthyroid approach. Author image.

cords are displayed and pre-procedure images recorded (Figure 9.5a). The tip of the vocal process is identified by palpation, and mobility of the cricoarytenoid joint is assessed. The chosen material is prepared and a suitable injection needle chosen. Some products have a compatible needle available (e.g. Radiesse Voice) which is long enough to reach the cords via the laryngoscope and is malleable. High viscosity implants (e.g. Bioplastique, fat) require a wider bore needle and use of a Brünings syringe to facilitate high-pressure injection. The needle must be primed with implant material at this stage to remove all air from the system.

The injection is placed lateral to the superior arcuate line, just anterior to the vocal process of the arytenoid cartilage (Point 'a' in Figure 9.6). The injection proceeds incrementally, observing the amount of medialization being achieved and watching carefully for extravasation or submucosal spread. If needed, more material can be injected a little more anteriorly (Point 'b' in Figure 9.6). The aim should be to produce a gently convex free edge of the cord reaching to the midline. Usually, a maximum of 0.3–0.4 ml is injected to reduce the possibility of airway obstruction. Gentle suction is used to remove any implant material which extrudes from the injection points and post-procedure images can then be recorded (Figure 9.5b shows the result of IL for a left vocal cord palsy).

Most patients can be treated on a day case basis, unless other comorbidities preclude this. There is little evidence that post-operative voice rest is of benefit, so the patient is simply advised to avoid excessive voice use for five to seven days. They should be warned that it might take several days for the benefits of the procedure to become established.

Local anaesthesia

LA procedures may be performed in an operating theatre, or an adequately equipped, staffed, and resourced outpatient setting. The patient is either seated

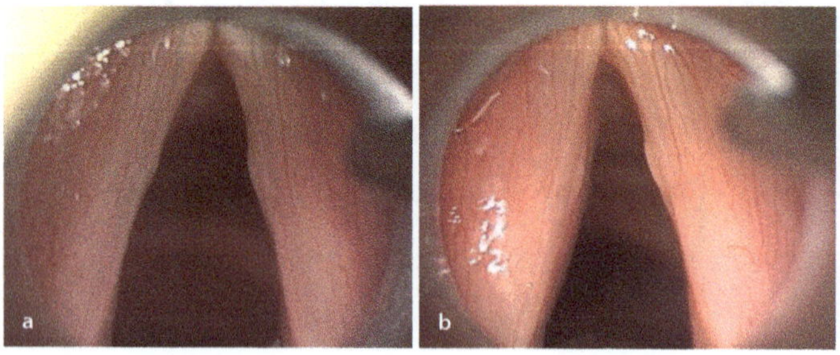

Figure 9.5: Left vocal cord palsy before IL (a) and after (b). Image courtesy Watson and Shaw.

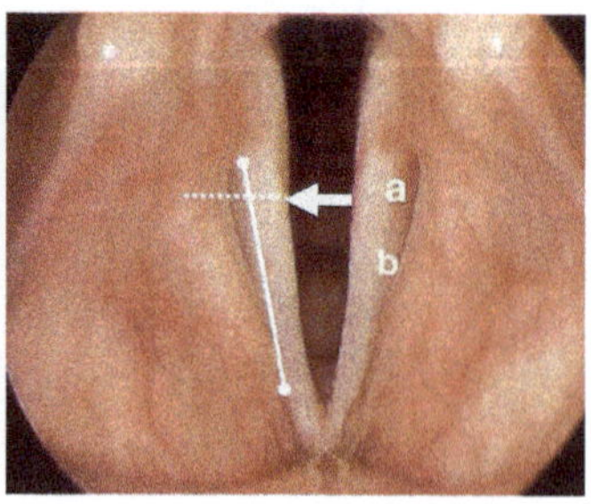

Figure 9.6: Site of injection. Image courtesy Watson and Shaw.

in a chair, or semi-recumbent on a couch. LA is delivered via several routes. Anaesthesia of the nose is needed if a flexible endoscope is to be used. This is administered via a nasal spray containing local anaesthetic and a vasoconstrictor. Mucosal anaesthesia of the larynx and pharynx can be delivered using 4% lignocaine via an ultrasonic nebuliser, or dripping the solution through a catheter directly into the larynx. For percutaneous approaches, local anaesthetic is also injected subcutaneously at the proposed injection site. If the transcricothyroid route is being used, a 'proof puncture' of the airway is easily performed at this point, with aspiration of tracheal air, and further LA can be directly injected into the lumen. Comprehensive local anaesthesia is fundamental to the achievement of success in these procedures and adequate time must be allowed for this.

Once the patient is anaesthetized and settled in a comfortable position, an assistant passes the flexible digital endoscope and displays a close-up view of the vocal cords on the monitor screen, which should be close to the patient's head so that the operator can easily see it. The implant should be prepared, along with a suitable needle.

Oral/transendoscopic approaches

For the oral route, a long malleable needle is used, as described earlier in the GA technique. For transendoscopic injections, a dedicated endoscopic injection system is needed. Once again, the needle must be primed with implant material to expel all air. The injection is placed in the vocal cord as in the GA technique. The injection is performed incrementally, and the patient can be asked to phonate to check that glottic closure has been achieved.

Percutaneous approaches

Transcricothyroid

The implant is prepared along with a 21G 50 mm needle, bent to an angle of approximately 45° and primed to remove air. The needle is passed through the cricothyroid membrane in the midline and visualized on the monitor screen (Figure 9.7a). It is directed toward the under surface of the vocal cord, a little anterior to the vocal process, and advanced through the conus elasticus into the thyroarytenoid muscle. The position of the needle tip can be demonstrated by gently 'jiggling' the needle from side to side at this stage. Injection once again proceeds incrementally (Figure 9.7b), with phonation to check progress until the desired result is obtained (Figure 9.7c). The patient can be asked to cough to help spread the material throughout thyroarytenoid. Care must be taken to ensure that the implant does not track into the subglottis, ventricle or false cord, or the submucosal plane. Rather more can be injected into the cord than in the GA technique, as the whole airway is visible during the procedure without hindrance from an endotracheal tube. Both cords can be injected during the same procedure for presbyphonia.

Transthyrohyoid

Once again, a primed 21G needle bent to 45° is used. It is passed in the midline almost vertically downward in the notch of the thyroid cartilage until the needle tip appears in the lumen next to the petiole of the epiglottis, just above the level of the vocal cords. It is then directed into position as for the GA technique, and injection proceeds as above.

Transthyroid

The thyroid ala is palpated on the side to be injected. The midpoint between the thyroid notch and the cricothyroid membrane is noted in the midline, and an imaginary line constructed between there and the posterior border of the ala. Injection is performed approximately half way along this line, with a straight, primed 21G needle. The needle passes through the cartilage and then a few millimetres into the thyroarytenoid. Once again, correct position can be confirmed by 'jiggling' the needle tip. Injection proceeds as for the transcricothyroid approach.

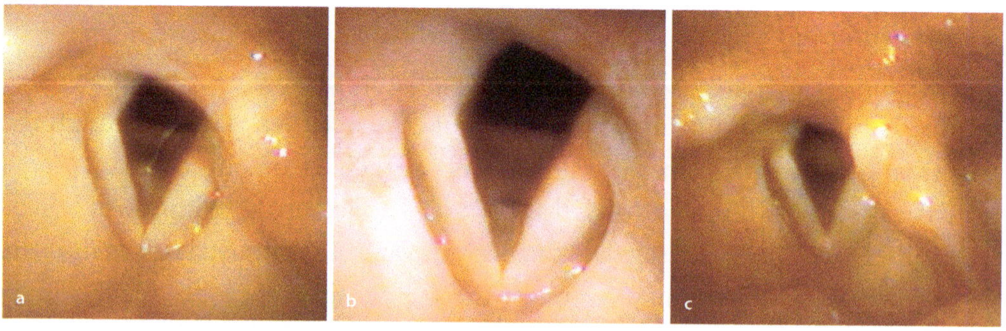

Figure 9.7: Transcricothyroid injection for left vocal cord palsy. Image courtesy Watson and Shaw. **a:** Needle position. **b:** Injection in progress. **c:** Left cord medialized.

After each of the LA techniques, the patient is observed for at least 30 minutes before being allowed to leave the unit, with strict instructions not to eat or drink for at least two hours until the LA has worn off. Once again, there is no evidence that voice rest is of benefit, but advice to avoid excessive voice use for five to seven days is given. It should be explained that it may take several days for the benefits of the IL to become apparent.

Follow up

Most patients have a telephone follow up with their speech therapist seven days after the procedure, to identify any problems and confirm that the patient is happy with the outcome. Residual dysphonia due to, for instance, an element of persisting supraglottic constriction may require further voice therapy.

Not all patients require formal clinic follow up. For patients with end of life diagnosis, if they are happy with the result, no further intervention is required. Those patients who have had a temporary implant can be asked to call the therapist as and when the improvement after IL has been lost.

Immediate post-operative advice and voice therapy

On the day patients are advised that:

- they should wait in ENT outpatients for 30 minutes after the procedure to ensure the airway remains patent – the surgeon will check each patient prior to departure from the hospital;
- they should not eat or drink for two hours or until the effects of the anaesthetic have subsided;
- they are free to cough, talk, and swallow as they need to;
- they may find small amounts of blood in their saliva and this is not a cause for concern;
- their throat is likely to feel sore once the anaesthetic has worn off, and possibly for several days after the procedure, and they should take painkillers as required; and
- no special modification of diet is required, but softer foods may be more comfortable initially.

Voice use for the first week

Patients are advised that:

- it may be necessary to take the following day off work and plan to avoid chairing meetings, telephone working, lecturing/teaching, etc., for the next five to seven days;
- the voice will sound different and, very often, worse for the first week;
- the voice/throat may feel different to use;
- they should use normal conversational voice for first week and avoid athletic vocal behaviours such as singing or shouting;
- they should try to reduce vocal effort levels as, now that glottic closure has been achieved, effortful laryngeal compensatory behaviours are no longer necessary; and
- the speech therapist will contact them by phone to review benefit from injection in one week.

Telephone review

- Therapist listens to voice quality and evaluates improvement in glottic closure and whether hyperfunctional compensatory behaviours are persisting or have resolved.
- GRBAS rating performed.
- Therapist asks patient's opinion on the improvement in voice quality, volume, vocal effort levels, comfort and shortness of breath during speech, etc.
- If patient and therapist agree that maximum expected benefit has been achieved, SLT advises patient to contact SLT when this benefit wears off, if the injection was a temporary implant material, or discharges the patient if the implant was a long-lasting implant material.
- If the therapist and patient agree that the result is suboptimal a further telephone review is arranged.
- If a suboptimal outcome persists the patient is offered a post-injection SLT consultation face-to-face: to trial therapy or to perform a further nasendoscopy to evaluate the reasons for the poor outcome.

Speech therapy management of suboptimal injection outcomes

- Most patients (90%) do not require further voice therapy after injection.
- If the voice remains aesthenic or breathy post-injection, it is likely that complete medialization has not been achieved, and a nasendoscopy may be beneficial to evaluate whether a top-up injection is more appropriate than voice therapy, or whether combining the improved post-injection proximity of the cords with voice therapy techniques will be enough to optimize the outcome to a satisfactory level. The types of voice therapy techniques which often deliver benefit in these circumstances are ones designed to maximize adduction without introducing cord lengthening, e.g. SOVT, Glottal strokes, Accent Method, etc.
- If the voice has become 'tight', strained, or rough (when it had not previously been so) it may be that too much injected material is present in the cord and that the cord is too turgid to support a mucosal wave. This is best evaluated under endoscopy and is unlikely to respond to voice therapy. The patient will need to be advised that the voice will improve as the temporary material is reabsorbed by the body. Regular telephone monitoring is recommended to allow the SLT to evaluate at what stage of reabsorption the voice is optimized, in order to advise ENT regarding estimating the level of reduction in the quantity of injected material in any future injections.
- If the voice was strained and rough prior to injection and remains so afterward, this may indicate that the patient is continuing to use the hyperfunctional supraglottic muscular compensation behaviours which had developed in response to the original glottal insufficiency (e.g. false cord constriction or A/P constriction). The patient may be continuing with these behaviours because the medialization was inadequate and glottic insufficiency persists, in which case a top-up injection may be necessary, or combining the improved post-injection vocal cord proximity with voice therapy as described above may be beneficial. Alternatively, medialization may be fully adequate but the patient may be struggling to 'let go' of these hyperfunctional muscular habits. In this case, therapy designed to reduce false cord constriction and effort reduction techniques may be effective (for example Voicecraft release of constriction, gentle hum, vocalized yawn, or Accent Method).

Complications and pitfalls

Major complications after IL are thankfully rare. Allergic reactions can occur to some biologically derived implants (e.g. bovine collagen). Haemorrhage or haematoma are possible, especially in those taking anticoagulants: avoid injection in this situation. Airway obstruction is rare. Patient intolerance of LA procedures is uncommon, even if they are anxious prior to the IL.

Tips and pearls

- Attend a course with animal or cadaver models to learn injection techniques.
- Become competent at GA IL at microlaryngoscopy first, before attempting LA approaches.
- Be willing to use different approaches for LA IL, dependent on the individual needs of the patient.
- Take time to provide sufficient local anaesthetic.
- Always site the implant at the level of the true vocal cord, deep to the ligament in thyroarytenoid.
- Do *not* inject Reinke's space.
- Do *not* inject patients taking anticoagulants.
- Do *not* produce over-medialization in the anterior part of the cord, which will produce a tight, strained voice quality.

Conclusion

IL is now a well-established technique for the management of glottal insufficiency. It can be performed easily under LA in an outpatient setting in many patients, and can be used at an early stage in the course of vocal fold palsy. Results following IL may be better in younger patients with a small posterior (as opposed to anterior) glottic gap. In many cases, IL can prevent the need for open surgical procedures such as type I thyroplasty.

Further reading

Arviso LC, Johns MM III, Mathison CC, Klein AM. 2010. Long-term outcomes of injection laryngoplasty in patients with potentially recoverable vocal fold paralysis. *Laryngoscope* **120**:2237–40.

Choi J, Son Y-I, So YK, et al. 2011. Posterior glottic gap and age as factors predicting voice outcome of injection laryngoplasty in patients with unilateral vocal fold paralysis. *J Laryngol Otol* **126**:260–6.

Damrose EJ. 2010. Percutaneous injection laryngoplasty in the management of acute vocal fold paralysis. *Laryngoscope* **120**:1582–90.

Brünings J. 1911. Uber eine neue Behandlungsmethode der Ranshlahmung. *Verhandl Ver Dtsh Laryngol* **18**:93–151.

Fang T-J, Li H-Y, Gliklitch RE, Chen Y-H, et al. 2010. Outcomes of fat injection laryngoplasty in unilateral vocal cord paralysis. *Arch Otolaryngol Head Neck Surg* **136**:457–62.

Friedman AD, Burns JA, Heaton JT, Zeitels SM. 2010. Early versus late injection medialization for unilateral vocal cord paralysis. *Laryngoscope* **120**:2042–6.

Kwon T-K, An S-Y, Ahn J-C, et al. 2010. Calcium hydroxylapatite injection laryngoplasty for the treatment of presbylaryngis: long-term results. *Laryngoscope* **120**:326–9.

Mathison CC, Villari CR, Klein AM, Johns MM III. 2009. Comparison of outcomes and complications between awake and asleep injection laryngoplasty: a case-control study. *Laryngoscope* **119**:1417–23.

Powell J, Carding P, Birdi R, Wilson JA. 2014. Injection laryngoplasty in the outpatient clinic under local anaesthetic: a case series of 68 patients. *Clin Otol* **39**:224–7.

Prendes BL, Yung KC, Kikhterov I, et al. 2012. Long-term effects of injection laryngoplasty with a temporary agent on voice quality and vocal fold position. *Laryngoscope* **122**:2227–33.

Tan M, Woo P. 2010. Injection laryngoplasty with micronized dermis: a 10-year experience with 381 injections in 344 patients. *Laryngoscope* **120**:2460–6.

Vinson KN, Zraick RI, Ragland FJ. 2010. Injection versus medialization laryngoplasty for the treatment of unilateral vocal fold paralysis: follow-up at 6 months. *Laryngoscope* **120**:1802–7.

Young VVN, Gartner-Schmidt J, Rosen CA. 2015. Comparison of voice outcomes after trial and long-term vocal fold augmentation in vocal fold atrophy. *Laryngoscope* **125**:934–940.

Young VVN, Smith LJ, Sulica L, et al. (2012) Patient tolerance of awake, in-office laryngeal procedures: a multi-institutional perspective. *Laryngoscope* **122**:315–21.

SECTION III: EXPANSION LARYNGOPLASTY

10

Type II thyroplasty: cordotomy and lateralization procedures

Simon Carney and Theodore Athanasiadis

Introduction

Whereas medialization procedures are most commonly performed for unilateral vocal fold immobility, lateralization procedures are almost invariably for bilateral fold immobility. The aim of surgery is to enlarge the airway whilst attempting to minimize any impact on vocal function and laryngeal competence although, in the words of Peter Belafsky: 'to surgically improve the glottic airway, one must typically "rob Peter to pay Paul"'.

Bilateral vocal fold immobility (BVFI) can be due to either bilateral fold paralysis or bilateral fold fixation. The latter can be due to fibrosis/stenosis of the cricoarytenoid joints or posterior glottic stenosis. Although microlaryngoscopy and probing can provide the surgeon with important information about the state of the cricoarytenoid joint, laryngeal electromyography (LEMG) is the optimal way to distinguish between paralysis and fixation and is essential if laryngeal reinnervation or laryngeal pacing is to be considered.

Tracheostomy remains a safe, albeit radical, technique to protect the airway while at the same time causing minimal impact on swallowing. One must accept that a tracheostomy does inhibit laryngeal elevation to a certain degree, along with vocal function. A fenestrated tube can be used if the larynx is competent in terms of secretion protection.

The following discussion aims to review the various surgical options for lateralizing the vocal fold(s) and will also address novel options, which may become mainstay treatments at some stage in the future.

Pathophysiology

When the recurrent laryngeal nerve is damaged, the vocal fold commonly sits in a paramedian position. Semon's law proposed that this was due to the muscular imbalance between a singular laryngeal abductor and several adductors. The Wagner–Grossmann hypothesis proposed that the observed fold position was actually due to the unopposed activity of the intact cricothyroid muscle. Through the use of LEMG, several authors have been able to disprove both of these theories. LEMG has established that the observed paramedian position is largely as a result of laryngeal synkinesis. There is also no doubt that paralysis of the vocal fold does cause secondary degenerative changes in the cricoarytenoid joints. This may explain many of the poor results that occur after laryngeal reinnovation procedures. Synkinesis has been demonstrated to be present in up to 88 % of all reinnervated vocal folds and remains a poor prognostic sign for good vocal fold mobility and function.

Many factors need to be taken into account when discussing the options of lateralization procedures with the patient. These include:

- medical comorbidities and drug history;
- age and suitability for general anaesthesia;
- the sensory status of the laryngeal mucosa;
- the social status of the patient and ability to manage a tracheostomy;
- occupation and vocal requirements;
- exercise tolerance and expectation;
- surgical expertise;
- adequate equipment; and
- financial resources.

Cordectomy/cordotomy

The terminology has changed over the years. The first description by Dennis and Kashima in 1991 described the procedure as a cordectomy, but cordotomy is now the preferred term as a result of subsequent modification of the technique. The surgical aim of simply 'releasing' the vocal fold (in contrast to the original description which was actually a partial resection of the glottis) is described. It is interesting that the term foldotomy has not been popularized now that laryngological nomenclature uses the term 'vocal fold' instead of 'vocal cord'.

The initial cordectomy was described as an excision of a C-shaped portion of the vocal fold just anterior to the vocal process, using a CO_2 laser. A cordotomy (Figure 10.1) involves a finer cut, perpendicular to the axis of the vocal cord just anterior to the vocal process, aimed to be a short, effective, and minimally invasive procedure. There remains controversy about whether one or both vocal folds should be treated in the first instance. There is no doubt that a bilateral procedure will improve the airway to a greater degree but that the risks of impaired vocal function are higher with an initial bilateral approach. Depending on the patient's airway and vocal requirements, most surgeons prefer to start with a single-sided procedure and then move on to the second vocal fold, if required, due to persistent airway restriction. If unilateral surgery is considered, the use of LEMG in the pre-operative phase may be extremely helpful in cases of asymmetry in terms of laryngeal innovation or synkinesis. If LEMG findings reveal no difference between the two sides, the vocal fold chosen will be purely upon surgical preference. It has been claimed that right-handed surgeons prefer operating on the left-hand side of the larynx but there is actually little evidence to support this presumption.

Amongst laryngologists, corticosteroids are used almost routinely in the peri-/post-operative period. Whereas elsewhere in the body, steroids have been demonstrated to decrease the amount of inflammation, granulation tissue, and scar formation, there are actually no prospective clinical trials to back this up with reference to laryngeal surgery. Nevertheless, when unexpected laryngeal oedema can cause rapid and significant airway obstruction, it would be prudent to minimize the risks as much as possible by using intra- and post-operative dexamethasone or equivalent intravenous steroid.

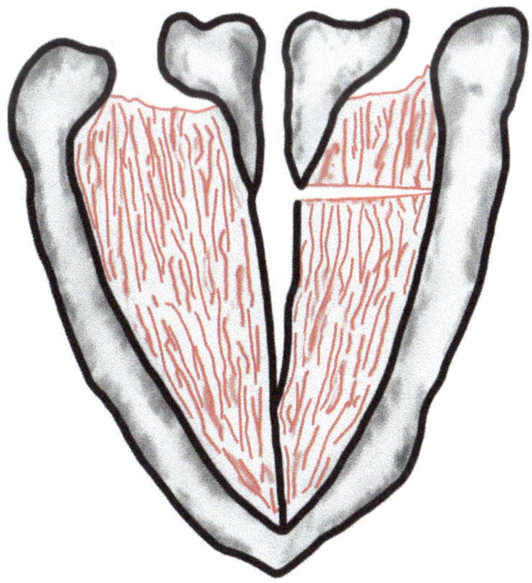

Figure 10.1: Location of posterior cordotomy of the left vocal cord. Author image.

Revision rates following cordotomy are variable in the published literature. Between 6% and 30% of patients have required more than one procedure in currently reported series, due to the formation of scar tissue in either the early or late post-operative period. More recently, radiofrequency plasma technology (Coblation© Laryngeal Wand: Smith & Nephew PLC, Austin, Texas) has been successfully used in place of the CO_2 laser. It is our experience that the natural healing properties of plasma, along with significantly less scar formation, make it ideal for revision surgery and also for selected primary bilateral cases due to its low cost, haemostasis, speed, and reduced risk of failure. Like all new techniques, however, its use remains controversial and there are many who still maintain that the CO_2 laser remains the instrument of choice.

Arytenoidectomy

In contrast to cordotomy, where the vocal process of the arytenoid is left intact, an arytenoidectomy aims to resect or ablate part or all of the arytenoid cartilage, including the vocal process (Figure 10.2). Thornell first described the first endoscopic arytenoidectomy in 1948. Ossoff then popularized the total arytenoidectomy technique in 1984. Crumley described a more conservative medial arytenoidectomy in 1993. A total arytenoidectomy involves the resection/ablation of at least the anterior two thirds of the arytenoid, whereas a medial arytenoidectomy aims to preserve at least two thirds of the arytenoid and focuses on removing the vocal process and the medial part of the main body in the posterior glottis (Figure 10.3), preserving the vibratory surface of the vocal fold whilst improving the posterior glottis airway. In contrast to cordotomy, the enhanced power and variable settings of the CO_2 laser allows this instrument to remain

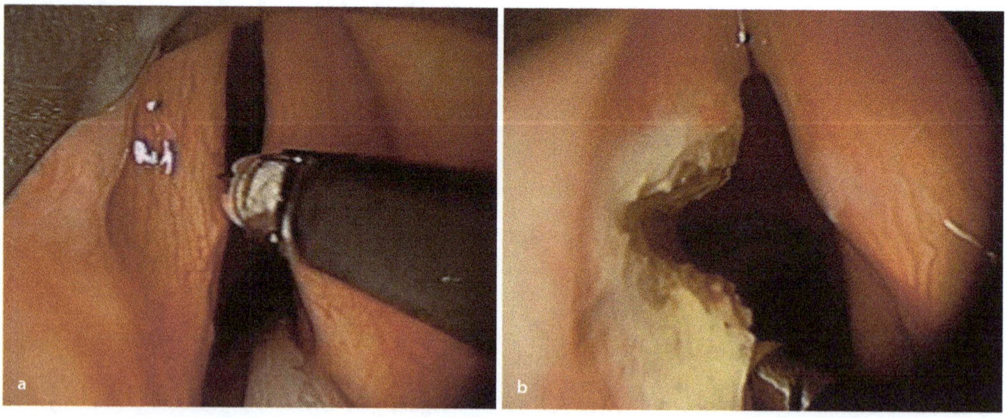

Figure 10.2: Coblation cordotomy. Left vocal fold, before (a) and after (b). Image courtesy of Carney.

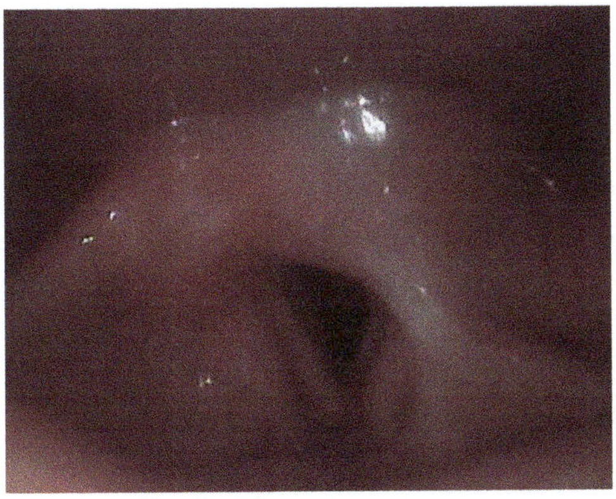

Figure 10.3: Arytenoidectomy – left; post-operative image. Author image.

as the current treatment of choice as plasma devices remain extremely slow in removing cartilage or ossified arytenoid tissue. Newer lasers with their advanced 'super-pulse' mode are able to deliver a precise cut at low temperatures, which greatly assists healing.

Up to a third of patients develop granulation tissue following arytenoidectomy, which can result in a significant decrease in airway patency. Current expert opinion would seem to favour more conservative arytenoidectomy given the high success rate, low rates of revision, and aspiration when compared to total arytenoidectomy. However, prospective randomized controls comparing these two techniques remain absent from the published literature.

Arytenoid abduction

Lateralization of the vocal fold (via forced abduction) can only be performed when the cricoarytenoid joint remains mobile. Proponents of the procedure claim that the theoretical attraction of arytenoid abduction (as opposed to more destructive airway procedures) is that forced abduction does not prevent the laryngeal adductors from acting during phonation and can therefore (theoretically at least) improve vocal function whilst providing a similar benefit in terms of an improved laryngeal airway. There is, however, little real physiological evidence to support this theory. Nevertheless, as the cricoarytenoid joint is a modified ball and socket joint, it is certainly true that fold abduction and expansion of the posterior glottis airway can be achieved by inferior traction of the muscular process and this alone validates arytenoid abduction as a surgical option.

The procedure is performed via an external approach with a skin incision being made in a transverse skin crease at the midpoint of the thyroid cartilage. The inferior constrictor muscle is divided at the posterior edge of the thyroid cartilage and the mucosa of the piriform fossa is bluntly dissected away from the cartilage until the posterior cricoarytenoid muscle is identified. This can then be followed posteriorly to the muscular process of the arytenoid. A permanent suture is then placed through the muscular process of the arytenoid and pulled inferiorly to result in abduction of the vocal fold. The desired position of the fold can be confirmed via flexible nasendoscopy. The suture is then secured to the inferior horn of the thyroid cartilage.

There is little in the way of reported case series in the literature. All series are small in number but report a high degree of success with less than 20% of patients experiencing any form of vocal dysfunction whatsoever. Case reports confirming its reversibility exist, where the suture has either snapped or been surgically removed with restoration of normal vocal fold function. There is no doubt that arytenoid abduction has a high learning curve and requires a high degree of surgical skill. The decision as to whether to perform abduction or an endoscopic airway-enlarging procedure will largely be determined by surgical training and expertise. In a patient where there is the potential for laryngeal recovery, the proven reversibility of the procedure means that arytenoid abduction can be an attractive non-destructive option in selected patients.

Suture lateralization

Suture lateralization is actually one of the earliest reported surgical techniques for vocal fold dysfunction. King first reported it in 1939 and the surgical aspects of the procedure have been refined significantly over the years with several dedicated instruments having been engineered to facilitate it as a minimally invasive option for patients who might not tolerate longer or more ablative procedures. With the advent of endolaryngeal suture instruments, only a tiny skin incision is required to bury the surgical knot and it has been reported that suture lateralization can be performed in combination with other airway enlarging procedures. A non-absorbable suture is passed through the laryngeal ventricle and out to the skin, then the distal end is looped around the vocal fold and passed out through the subglottis and cricothyroid membrane so that the thread forms a loop around the vocal process. A second suture between the anterior third and the middle third has also been described as a technical variant to further improve the laryngeal airway. This more anterior second suture causes more vocal dysfunction and should be reserved for selected resistant cases. There is no doubt that this simple technique does significantly improve the laryngeal airway. In reported series, although good results are initially reported, the vocal fold often medializes over time, probably due to suture migration. However, in some patients, successful results of up to five years have been reported. Initial dysphonia exists in a much higher proportion of patients than with ablative procedures but this does improve with vocal rehabilitation. See Chapter 3 on speech therapy.

The advantages of suture lateralization are that it is a quick procedure and is also potentially reversible. Its disadvantages are the high rates of early dysphonia and increasing failure rates over time.

Laryngeal reinnervation

With confirmed transection of the recurrent laryngeal nerves, where there is little chance for recovery, laryngeal reinnervation has emerged as an innovative technique in the armamentarium of the laryngologist. Both 'unselective' and 'selective' reinnervation techniques have been reported; in the latter, selected muscle groups are reinnervated as opposed to the whole recurrent laryngeal nerve itself. Unselective reinnervation has been reported mainly for unilateral vocal fold paralysis where the sole aim has been to improve the tone and bulk of the paralysed laryngeal muscles. In bilateral vocal fold paresis (where the cricoarytenoid joints are confirmed to be mobile), selective reinnervation of the posterior cricoarytenoid muscle is designed to selectively trigger vocal fold abduction during the inspiratory phase of respiration.

The earliest reports of selective reinnervation used a pedicle of omohyoid muscle along with its branch of the ansa cervicalis nerve, implanted into the posterior cricoarytenoid muscle. The use of the phrenic nerve has now attracted considerable attention. The phrenic nerve is an attractive conduit due to its motor neurones being active during inspiration. Unilateral phrenic nerve division has been demonstrated to cause little impairment of diaphragmatic movement and a unilateral phrenic nerve can be split and used to reinnervate both sides of the larynx. This greatly simplifies the surgical procedure.

There are a few case reports claiming successful laryngeal reinnervation but the literature remains devoid of large prospective series or randomized controlled trials. Animal studies provide the greatest source of evidence thus far, but these techniques should still be regarded as experimental and only of consideration in the young, fit, and informed patient, where there is a high expectation in terms of future vocal function and exercise expectations.

Laryngeal pacing

Selective pacing of the abductor muscles was first successfully performed in pigs, and early series in humans are now being reported. In a similar philosophy to hypoglossal nerve stimulation for obstructive sleep apnoea, an implant is placed in the intercostal muscles, which detects the inspiratory phase of respiration and provides electrical stimulation to the peripheral branches of the recurrent laryngeal nerve servicing the abductor muscles. The early clinical results of hypoglossal nerve stimulation have proven to be better than previously imagined and, similarly, the most recent research (albeit non-controlled) suggests unilateral laryngeal pacing is superior to unilateral cordotomy in selected patients. While it is too early to make any bold claims about this procedure, it is highly likely that laryngeal pacing will become an active area for both basic science and clinical research over the next few years.

Botulinum toxin

Because of our emerging understanding on how laryngeal synkinesis prevents optimal outcomes following fold paralysis, the use of botulinum toxin (Botox) to reduce its impact is certainly logical. The aim is to selectively eliminate the activity of the thyroarytenoid and lateral cricoarytenoid muscles, allowing for unopposed posterior cricoarytenoid activity and resulting vocal fold abduction. The success of botulinum toxin in spasmodic dysphonia has stimulated interest in using it to prevent synkinesis and the first report of using it in a patient with bilateral vocal fold paralysis demonstrated an improvement in peak flow rates over a two-year period. Subsequent to this, several small case series have emerged in the literature. Fine-wire LEMG has emerged as a technique that can potentially identify areas of synkinesis, which could potentially be targeted by botulinum toxin. Nevertheless, the lack of long term benefit (the procedure needs to be repeated at least every three months) and limited clinical outcomes when compared to other procedures leads us to conclude that selective botulinum toxin injection can only be regarded as an adjunct procedure to be used in combination with the other surgical methods reported in this chapter.

Summary and conclusions

In cases of bilateral vocal fold immobility, the selection of an appropriate lateralization procedure should be determined by the exact diagnosis, prognosis for recovery, and appropriate patient surgical factors.

The 'robbing Peter to pay Paul' philosophy should remain paramount in the surgeon's mind at all times. In our opinion, irrespective of diagnosis, if rapid airway improvement is the critical requirement to achieve decannulation or avoidance of a tracheostomy, endoscopic procedures such as bilateral cordotomy or medial arytenoidectomy remain the surgical treatments of choice. In cases of bilateral fold paralysis where there is the possibility of laryngeal recovery, although cordotomy/medial arytenoidectomy remain as safe and effective options, suture lateralization or arytenoid abduction emerge as surgical alternatives. The use of LEMG, where available, can help the multidisciplinary voice team distinguish between laryngeal muscle paralysis and fold fixation. If the cricoarytenoid joints are fibrosed or ankylosed, then arytenoid abduction or suture lateralization are likely to be ineffective and cordotomy/medial arytenoidectomy are the treatments of choice.

Future research directed at laryngeal reinnervation and laryngeal pacing give the authors optimism that in the future, partial or total recovery of vocal fold function will be achievable for many more patients with bilateral vocal fold paralysis.

Further reading

Applebaum EL, Allen GW, Sisson GA. 1979. Human laryngeal reinnervation: the Northwestern experience. *Laryngoscope* **89**:1784–7.

Aubry K, Leboulanger N, Harris R, et al. 2010. Laser arytenoidectomy in the management of bilateral vocal cord paralysis in children. *Int J Pediatr Otorhi* **74**:451–5.

Bajaj Y, Sethi N, Shayah A, et al. 2009. Vocal fold paralysis: role of bilateral transverse cordotomy. *J Laryngol Otol* **123**:1348–51.

Belafsky PC. 2011. Bilateral vocal fold immobility. *Curr Opin Otolaryngol* **19**:415.

Blitzer A, Jahn AF, and Keidar A. 1996. Semon's law revisited: an electromyographic analysis of laryngeal synkinesis. *Ann Otol Rhinol Laryn* 105:764–9.

Bizakis JG, Papadakis CE, Karatzanis AD, et al. 2004. The combined endoscopic CO(2) laser posterior cordectomy and total arytenoidectomy for treatment of bilateral vocal cord paralysis. *Clin Otolaryngol Allied Sci* **29**:51–4.

Bosley B, Rosen CA, Simpson CB, et al. 2005. Medial arytenoidectomy versus transverse cordotomy as a treatment for bilateral vocal fold paralysis. *Ann Otol Rhinol Laryn* **114**:922–6.

Chan CL, Frauenfelder CA, Foreman A, et al. 2015. Surgical management of airway stenosis by radiofrequency coblation. *J Laryngol Otol* **129** Suppl 1:S21–S26.

Crumley RL. 2000. Laryngeal synkinesis revisited. *Ann Oto Rhinol Laryn* **109**:365–71.

Crumley RL. 1993. Endoscopic laser medial arytenoidectomy for airway management in bilateral laryngeal paralysis. *Ann Oto Rhinol Laryn* **102**:81–4.

Damrose EJ. 2011. Suture laterofixation of the vocal fold for bilateral vocal fold immobility. *Curr Opin Otolaryngo* **19**:416–21.

Dennis DP, and Kashima H. 1989. Carbon dioxide laser posterior cordectomy for treatment of bilateral vocal cord paralysis. *Ann Oto Rhinol Laryn* **98**:930–4.

Koufman JA, Walker FO, and Joharji GM. 1995. The cricothyroid muscle does not influence vocal fold position in laryngeal paralysis. *Laryngoscope* **105**:368–72.

Marina MB, Marie JP, and Birchall MA. 2011. Laryngeal reinnervation for bilateral vocal fold paralysis. *Curr Opin Otolaryngo* **19**:434–8.

Mueller AH. Laryngeal pacing for bilateral vocal fold immobility. 2011. *Curr Opin Otolaryngo* 19:439–43.

Muller A, and Paulsen FP. 2002. Impact of vocal cord paralysis on cricoarytenoid joint. *Ann Oto Rhinol Laryn* **111**:896–901.

Nawka T, Sittel C, Gugatschka M, et al. 2015. Permanent transoral surgery of bilateral vocal fold paralysis: A prospective multi-center trial. *Laryngoscope* **125**:1401–8.

Ongkasuwan J, and Courey M. 2011. The role of botulinum toxin in the management of airway compromise due to bilateral vocal fold paralysis. *Curr Opin Otolaryngo* **19**:444–8.

Ossoff RH, Sisson GA, Duncavage JA, et al. 1984. Endoscopic laser arytenoidectomy for the treatment of bilateral vocal cord paralysis. *Laryngoscope* **94**:1293–7.

Quiney RE, and Michaels L. 1990. Histopathology of vocal cord palsy from recurrent laryngeal nerve damage. *J Otolaryngol* **19**:237–241.

Sapundzhiev N, Lichtenberger G, Eckel HE, et al. 2008. Surgery of adult bilateral vocal fold paralysis in adduction: history and trends. *Eur Arch Oto-Rhino-L* **265**:1501–14.

Thornell WC. 1949. A new intralaryngeal approach in arytenoidectomy in bilateral abductor paralysis of the vocal cords; report of three cases. *Arch Otolaryngol* **50**:634–9, illust.

Vilensky JA, and Sinish PR. 2004. Sir Felix Semon and Semon's law. *Clin Anat* **17**:605–6.

Young VN, and Rosen CA. 2011. Arytenoid and posterior vocal fold surgery for bilateral vocal fold immobility. *Curr Opin Otolaryngo* **19**:422–7.

SECTION IV: RELAXING

11

Type III relaxation thyroplasty: midline wedge

Vyas Prasad and Marc Remacle

Isshiki described the type III thyroplasty primarily for patients requiring pitch lowering not amenable or responsive to conservative or medical intervention.

Conditions requiring relaxation thyroplasty (type III)

The main groups are:

- female-to-male transsexual patients:
  - not fully responsive to or unhappy with results of androgen therapy;
- mutational falsetto (puberphonia) mainly in males:
  - failure of voice therapy,
  - failure of psychotherapy, or
  - failure of Botox treatment to the cricothyroid muscle; and
- high-pitched dysphonia:
  - breathy voice,
  - narrow glottic chink, or
  - small amplitude of vibration (stiff cord).

Assessment process, baseline measurements, and pre-work up

History – mutational falsetto

Patients with a history of mutational falsetto or puberphonia should have any underlying endocrinological cause excluded prior to embarking on medical or surgical intervention.

A thorough history should include identifying the following details:

- vocal impairment:
  - hoarseness,
  - breathiness,
  - shallow breathing,
  - muscle tension,
  - lack of pitch variability,
  - voice weakness;
- psychological/psychosocial issues:
  - embarrassment with 'new voice',
  - failure to accept adulthood,
  - over identification with maternal figure,
  - social immaturity,
  - desire to maintain 'soprano' singing voice;
- previous or current treatment:
  - voice therapy,
  - psychotherapy,
  - Botox therapy; and
- endocrine history:
  - thyroid disease,
  - secondary sexual characteristics.

Clinical examination

In addition to a full ENT examination and a fibreoptic nasendoscopy and laryngoscopy, we recommend videolaryngostroboscopy (VLS) with recording facilities for pre-operative documentation. The ENT surgeon should at the very least ask the patient about secondary sexual characteristics if they are not examined for them.

Voice assessment

Vocal function is evaluated according to the protocol recommended by the Committee on Phoniatrics of the European Laryngological Society. This is a multidimensional set of minimal basic measurements suitable for all 'common' dysphonias. It consists of five different aspects:

- perception (grade, roughness, breathiness);
- videostroboscopy (closure, regularity, mucosal wave and symmetry);
- acoustics (jitter, shimmer, F0-range and softest intensity);
- aerodynamics (phonation quotient); and
- subjective rating (Voice Handicap Index – VHI, Visual Analogue Scale – VAS).

The lowering of pitch when pressure is applied to the anterior thyroid cartilage backwards during phonation (manual or Gutzmann's test) should lower the pitch and may predict success from relaxation thyroplasty.

Treatment options and consent

The management of patients with mutational falsetto, or transsexuals who require further pitch lowering, is multidisciplinary. Patients with mutational falsetto usually improve with voice therapy and/or psychotherapy. The later the therapy is initiated, the less likely its success. In transsexuals, however, the perceived or objective lack of response to androgen therapy affecting these individuals usually obviates the need for non-surgical treatments.

Non-surgical options

- Voice therapy.
- Psychotherapy.
- Botox injection to cricothyroid (short-term).

Surgical options

- Open.
- Laryngeal framework surgery:
  - Isshiki type III thyroplasty;
  - Tucker's modification thyroplasty;
  - Kocak's modification thyroplasty (window relaxation);
  - Modified Isshiki type IIIB (relaxation thyroplasty – Figure 11.1).

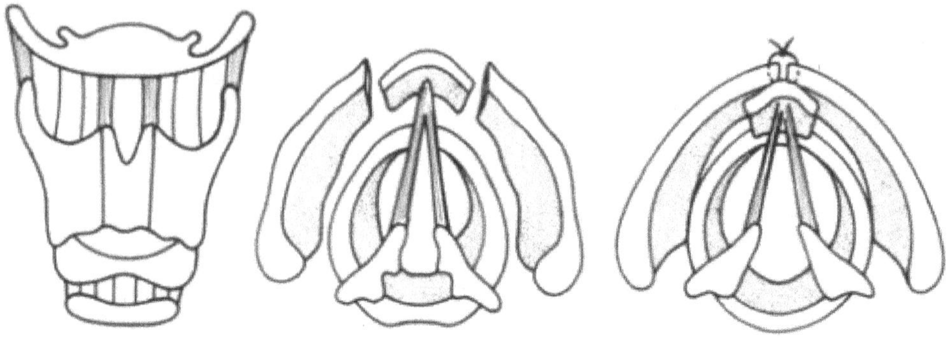

Figure 11.1: Schematic diagram of relaxation thyroplasty type IIIB. Image courtesy of Remacle.

Consent

All patients undergoing surgery should be counselled appropriately about the benefits and risks of having the procedure. The potential of not having the procedure, the pros and cons, and the alternatives (surgical or medical), as well as the possibility of conservative management. This may potentially be the best option (informed consent) and should be discussed. The type of anaesthesia, length of stay, peri-operative care, and post-operative course should be made known in simple and clear language to avoid unnecessary anxiety or misunderstanding. The multidisciplinary nature of treatment should be emphasized from the start, with good access to the voice therapist throughout the patient pathway.

In the modified type III, i.e. IIIB thyroplasty, we counsel all patients on general operative risks, including those involving either local or general anaesthesia, pain, bleeding, and infection. Specific risks of the procedure include airway compromise and dyspnoea, minor extra-laryngeal haematoma, breach after dissection into the laryngeal lumen, and worsening of voice both immediately after or later which may still require further speech (voice) therapy input.

Operative procedure

Step 1 – Anaesthesia

Patients are given the option of having either a local anaesthetic with sedation and analgesia administered intravenously, or a general anaesthetic. Monitored anaesthetic care (MAC) during local anaesthesia is now more commonly performed in this setting. The benefits of local anaesthesia are that we can assess pitch lowering with the patient phonating (usually with the vowel /a/).

Local anaesthesia (LA)

- Intravenous opioid for pain control – remifentanyl.
- Intravenous benzodiazepine for amnesis and anxiolysis – midazolam.
- Intravenous short acting sedative and hypnotic – propofol.
- Anticholinergic – glycopyrrolate to reduce secretions.
- Local anaesthesia injection to operative site and trachea – lignocaine 1% with 1:200,000 adrenaline.
- Intravenous antibiotics pre-operatively.
- Intravenous corticosteroid pre-operatively.
- Oxygen administered via face mask.
- Cardiopulmonary monitoring check complements anaesthetic chapter.

General anaesthesia (GA)

- Laryngeal mask airway (LMA) preferred over size 6 endotracheal tube (Figure 11.2).
- Transnasal fibreoptic videoendoscopy through LMA.
- Assessment of anterior commissure retrusion.

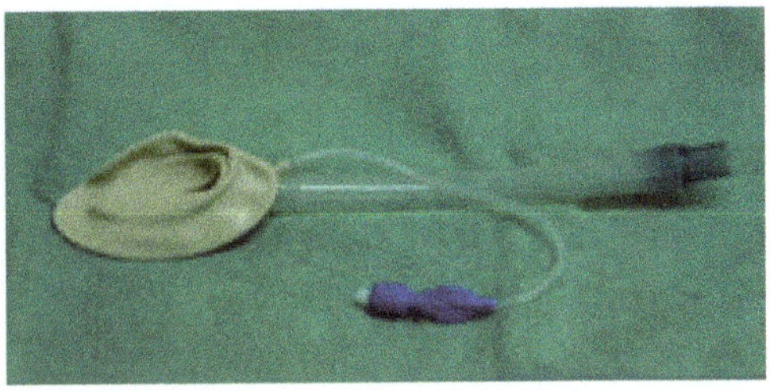

Figure 11.2: Laryngeal mask airway (LMA). Image courtesy of Remacle.

Step 2 – Positioning

All patients are positioned supine with slight extension of the neck. In LA cases, the face is not covered so as to allow for interaction with the patient during assessment of phonation after retrusion of the anterior cartilage segment. A drape is placed on the patient's chin and secured over two intravenous drip stands either side of the patient's head (Figure 11.3).

Step 3 – Specific equipment

Besides a fine-cut side-end cutting burr or oscillating sagittal saw to make the vertical cuts in the thyroid cartilage, we use quick setting Tissucol fibrin glue (Immuno AG, Baxter®, Deerfield, IL, USA) over the displaced anterior segment to help with haemostasis and cover any potential breaches in the inner perichondrium.

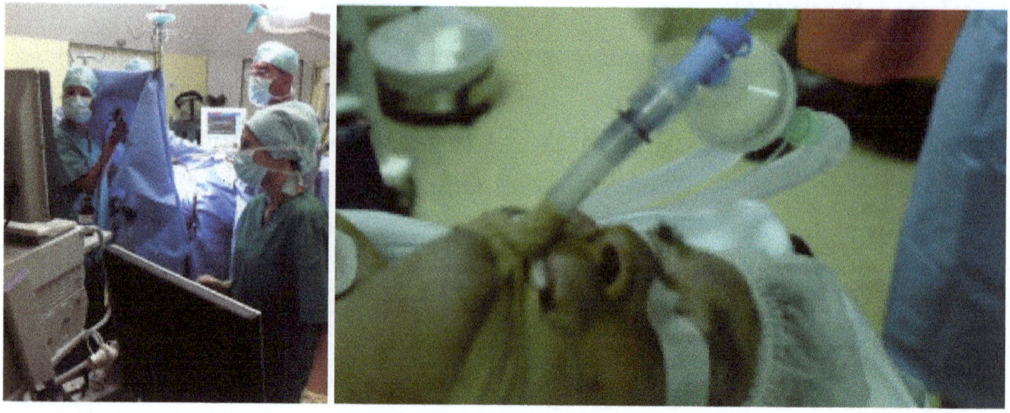

Figure 11.3: Left: operating theatre setup under LA. Right: patient under GA using LMA. Images courtesy of Remacle.

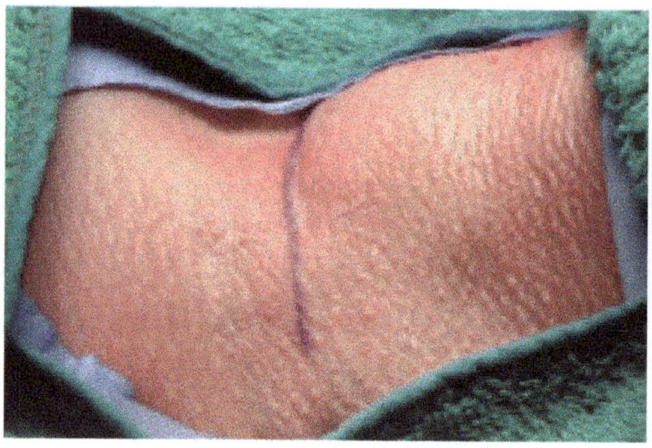

Figure 11.4: Neck prepared with skin marking (patient's head positioned at 3 o'clock). Image courtesy of Remacle.

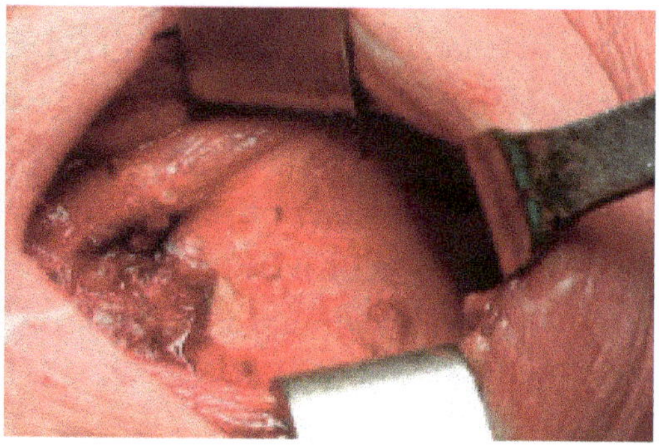

Figure 11.5: Exposure of thyroid cartilage. Image courtesy of Remacle.

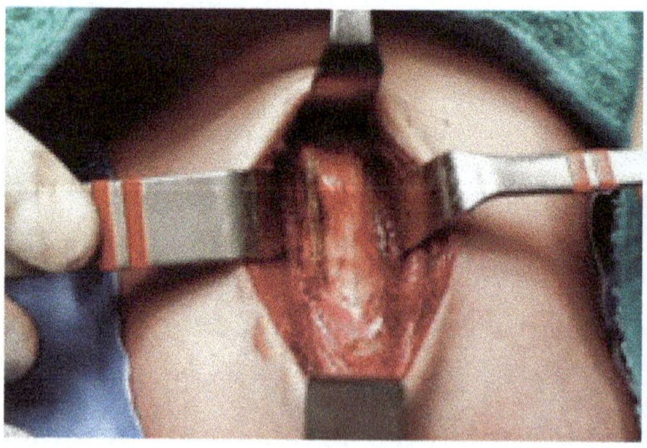

Figure 11.6: Vertical incisions either side of midline (patient's head situated at 12 o'clock). Image courtesy of Remacle.

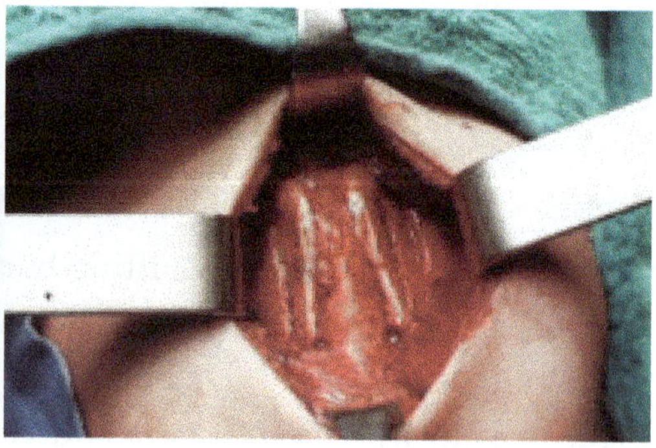

Figure 11.7: Separation of anterior segment and elevation of inner perichondrium (patient's head positioned at 12 o'clock). Image courtesy of Remacle.

Step 4 – Incision and raising of flaps

After the patient is prepared and draped in a sterile setting, a horizontal midline incision approximately 4 cm long, and preferably in a neck crease, is made (Figure 11.4).

Subplatysmal flaps are raised and the deep investing layer of cervical fascia is identified and cut. The strap muscles are retracted laterally and the thyroid cartilage is exposed on both sides with adequate view of at least 1 cm either side of the midline in its entire length, i.e. both superior and inferior margins (Figure 11.5).

Step 5 – Incising the thyroid cartilage

Vertical incisions 5 mm either side of the midline are made from the superior down to the inferior rim of the thyroid cartilage (Figure 11.6). The landmarks used for the formation of the window are the thyroid notch and the inferior border of the thyroid cartilage. Calcified cartilage is cut using the fine side-end burr, or a sagittal saw. The cuts extend through the outer perichondrium and thyroid cartilage without extending through the inner perichondrium.

The anterior 1 cm of the inner perichondrium is carefully elevated from the posterior cartilage segment bilaterally using an angled elevator. The anterior cartilage segment with attached Broyle's ligament is retrodisplaced into the larynx and the posterior segments are allowed to override it on either side laterally (Figure 11.7).

Step 6 – Endoscopic evaluation and closure

An endoscope is either passed through the patient's nose (LA) or the LMA (GA) and the degree of retrusion noted, as well as any internal laryngeal breach. The segments of the thyroid cartilage lateral toof the anterior segment are secured in position over the middle segment with 3-0 nylon sutures (Figure 11.8).

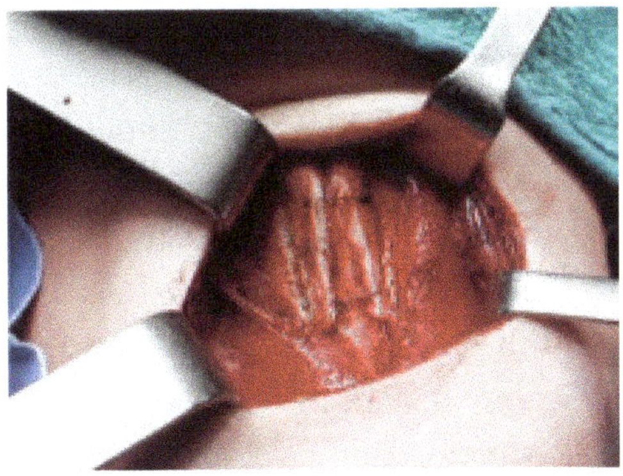

Figure 11.8: Segments of thyroid cartilage secured in position (patient's head positioned at 12 o'clock). Image courtesy of Remacle.

The wound is closed in layers after the application of fibrin glue over the retrusion site and insertion of a small suction drain.

Post-operative advice and voice therapy

Patients are advised a week of low-intensity voicing after discharge and placed on a 5-day course of broad-spectrum oral antibiotics, steroid inhalers, and proton-pump inhibitors empirically. All patients undergo voice therapy after surgery to optimize the functional results with the new glottic configuration. We follow the recommendations of the Committee of Phoniatrics of the European Laryngological Society (ELS) for voice assessment.

Patients are reviewed in the voice clinic setting a week after the procedure to check on the wound and voice. Thereafter, they are reviewed regularly at six to eight weekly intervals until their voice has been fully optimized.

Common pitfalls/mistakes

- Surgery for mutational falsetto undertaken too early without adequate speech therapy.
- Inadequate counselling of the benefit of type IIIB thyroplasty in cases of stiff vocal cords with a narrow chink. Therefore, a possible need to combine the procedure with medialization thyroplasty type I.
- The vertical incisions made too deep, resulting in breach of the inner perichondrium of the thyroid cartilage.

Tips and pearls

- Speech and psychotherapy should not be delayed in cases of mutational falsetto as failure of conservative therapy is more likely.
- Type IIIB thyroplasty should be considered the preferred permanent treatment of choice in mutational falsetto, and can be recommended in cases where transsexuals are unhappy with androgen therapy (female to male).
- In scarred or stiff vocal cords secondary to laryngeal trauma, radiation, chronic laryngitis, sulcus vocalis, and vocal cord atrophy, a type IIIB procedure may be of benefit, although results are less favourable compared with surgery for mutational falsetto.

Further reading

Dagli M, Sati I, Acar A, et al. 2008. Mutational falsetto: intervention outcomes in 45 patients. *J Laryngol Otol* **122**:277–81.

Dejonckere PH, Bradley P, Clemente P, et al. 2001. A basic protocol for functional assessment of voice pathology, especially for investigating the efficacy of (phonosurgical) treatments and evaluating new assessment techniques. Guideline elaborated by the Committee on Phoniatrics of the European Laryngological Society (ELS). *Eur Arch Otorhinolaryngol* **258**:77–82.

Isshiki N. 1989. *Phonosurgery: Theory and Practice.* Tokyo: Springer.

Isshiki N, Taira T, Tanabe M. 1988. Surgical treatment for vocal pitch disorders. In: Fujimora O. (ed) *Vocal Physiology: Voice Productions, Mechanisms and Functions.* New York, NY: Raven Press, pp. 449–58.

Kaplan SL. 1982. Mutational falsetto. *J Am Acad Child Psychiatry* **21**:82–5.

Kocak I, Dogan M, Tadihan E, et al. 2008. Window anterior commissure relaxation laryngoplasty in the management of high-pitched voice disorders. *Arch Otolaryngol Head Neck Surg* **134**:1263–9.

Li GD, Mu L, Yang S. 1999. Acoustic evaluation of Isshiki type III thyroplasty for treatment of mutational voice disorders. *J Laryngol Otol* **113**:31–4.

Soderplan E, Larsson AK, Almquist SA. 2004. Evaluation of a conservative group of transsexual individuals referred for vocal intervention in the west of Sweden. *Logoped Phoniatr Vocol* **29**:18–30.

Tucker HM. 1985. Anterior commissure laryngoplasty for adjustment of vocal fold tension. *Ann Otol Rhinol Laryngol* **94**:547–9.

SECTION V: TENSING

12

Type IV thyroplasty: cricothyroid approximation

Meredydd Harries and Declan Costello

Introduction

Laryngeal framework surgery (LFS) is defined as surgery that involves an external approach to the laryngeal skeleton to change the position, length, mass or tension of the vocal folds. Isshiki classified LFS into different types, and cricothyroid approximation is also known as a type IV thyroplasty.

Cricothyroid approximation (CA) increases the pitch or fundamental frequency of the voice by simulating the action of the cricothyroid muscle with sutures.

The paired cricothyroid muscles are located at the front of the larynx and are the only intrinsic muscles of the larynx that are located outside the cartilaginous framework. Their motor innervation comes from the external branch of the superior laryngeal nerve, which again is different from the other intrinsic laryngeal muscles (which are supplied by the recurrent laryngeal nerve). The human cricothyroid muscle comprises three bellies: rectus, oblique, and horizontal. Many clinicians and researchers have considered their muscle type and innervation patterns and suggested different actions for each, including phonatory and respiratory functions. In spite of this, there appears to be no common consensus. The rectus belly may be more involved in the fast change of pitch during speech articulation whereas the oblique belly may determine slower changes at higher frequencies. These different properties have lead to some experiments with different suture positions for CA surgery but these have not been conclusive or widely adopted.

Indications

To raise the fundamental frequency of the voice and, hence, vocal pitch.

1. Cricothyroid muscle paralysis is difficult to diagnose clinically and its effect on the voice is subtle. It may be unilateral or bilateral.
2. Cricothyroid approximation is used in transgender voice feminization surgery and, therefore, is commonly performed with a thyroid chondroplasty ('thyroid shave'). This brings the pitch of the voice closer to the female range and loses the male thyroid cartilage protuberance.
3. Cricothyroid approximation could also be considered in managing patients with androphonia where medical treatment has failed. This chapter will not go into detail on the thyroid shave. However, it should be noted that it is essential to avoid over-resection of the thyroid cartilage. The anterior commissure lies at a point halfway down the thyroid cartilage; it is essential that this midpoint of the thyroid cartilage anteriorly is not breached as this can lead to detachment of the anterior commissure. In this situation, both vocal folds lose tension, resulting in lowering of the pitch as well as other voice problems.

Patient selection and pre-operative care

Patients undergoing male-to-female gender reassignment (transgender) will frequently identify their voice as being a limiting factor in achieving a satisfactory transition. Feminization of voice relies not only on pitch elevation, but also on alteration of consonant production and on speech inflection. For this reason, before pitch-raising surgery is considered, the patient should be assessed and treated by a specialist speech and language therapist (SLT) with an interest in voice disorders, and with experience in working with transgender patients. The SLT needs to consider all features of feminization of the voice, not just pitch. It can be useful to record measures of fundamental frequency to monitor pitch-raising, both achieved through therapy and through surgery.

Procedure

This may be undertaken using a general or local anaesthetic as the surgeon or patient prefers. Much has been made of the fact that LFS carried out under local anaesthesia has the advantage of auditory feedback and, whereas this is true for medialization procedures, for CA this may not be so important. The authors prefer general anaesthesia as the technique described below involves tying the sutures as tightly as possible and does not use auditory feedback from the patient's voice to alter the suture positions or tension.

The patient is positioned with the neck extended. Local anaesthetic with adrenaline is infiltrated into the incision to reduce bleeding and give some pain relief in the immediate post-operative period.

The incision is made at the lower border of the thyroid cartilage, extending from the midline to the oblique line of the thyroid cartilage – which is around 3–4 cm on either side. Subcutaneous flaps are raised and the thyroid and cricoid cartilage palpated. The cricothyroid artery runs horizontally at the lower border of the thyroid cartilage and should be avoided or cauterized early in the procedure.

The strap muscles can usually be retracted laterally and the cricothyroid muscle exposed (Figure 12.1).

Removal of the muscle does improve the exposure of the cartilages and can facilitate the suture insertion but we would try to keep the muscle in situ to preserve any residual function that could improve the approximation at a later stage. At this stage the distance between the cricoid and the thyroid cartilages can be observed (Figure 12.1).

Traditionally, four sutures are placed between the cartilages. The cricoid is usually soft enough for the sutures to be inserted and it is important for all four sutures to be inserted before moving on to the thyroid cartilage. There are different recommendations for the type of material used, such as nylon or silk, or even wires. We would use a nonabsorbable material such as a 2-0 silk on a cutting needle, but it is very much the surgeons' choice and no material has been

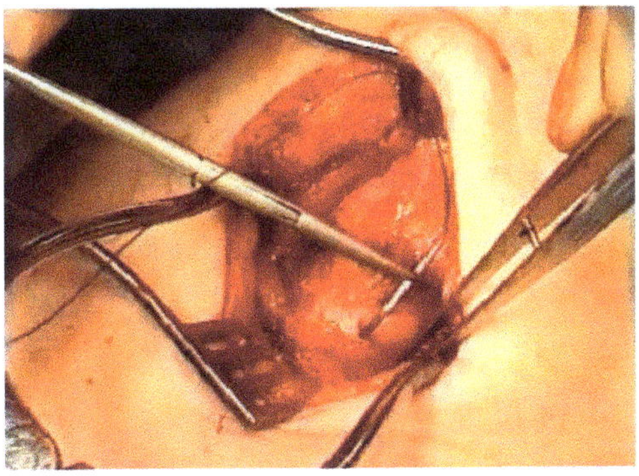

Figure 12.1: Note the large distance between the cricoid and thyroid cartilage. Author image.

shown to be superior. The cricoid sutures are placed at the midline and 0.5 cm laterally on either side.

It is important to avoid breaching the inner mucosal surface as this can lead to irritation and granulation tissue within the subglottis.

The sutures should be retracted inferiorly to allow unobstructed access to the thyroid cartilage superiorly.

The thyroid cartilage is usually too hard to pass the suture through without risk of fracture of the lamina, especially anteriorly where the lamina is thinnest. We use a drill to make four holes, each 0.5 cm above its inferior border – 0.5 cm to the midline and the other a further 0.5cm laterally on each side. A periosteal elevator can be used to protect the inner perichondrium of the thyroid cartilage and prevent damage to the medial laryngeal structures.

The positioning of the sutures is important as the pitch raising effect seems to be best when mimicking the action of the rectus belly of the muscle, so the more anterior the sutures the better (Figure 12.2).

Once all four sutures are in place they can be tied as tightly as possible in our practice (Figures 12.3 and 12. 5). The medial sutures are tied first and then each lateral suture. Other authors have described the use of different types of bolsters (Figures 12.4 and 12. 6) or protection to prevent the sutures from cutting through the cartilage and to possibly give better long term results by preventing loosening with time. Closure is with 4-0 vicryl for deep sutures and a 5-0 prolene to skin. We do not routinely insert a drain or give antibiotics.

A light dressing over the wound is sufficient and the procedure is performed as a day case with the patient able to leave hospital within six hours from the end of the operation.

Complications

These may include wound infection, haemorrhage, haematoma, pain, and scarring, as with any open procedure. Specific complications include a reduction in the range of the voice and a strained quality to the voice.

Results

It is important to be realistic as to what this procedure can do to the voice.

For cricothyroid paralysis the results can be very good in both the short and long term as the underlying problem is a loss of tension. Unilateral procedures

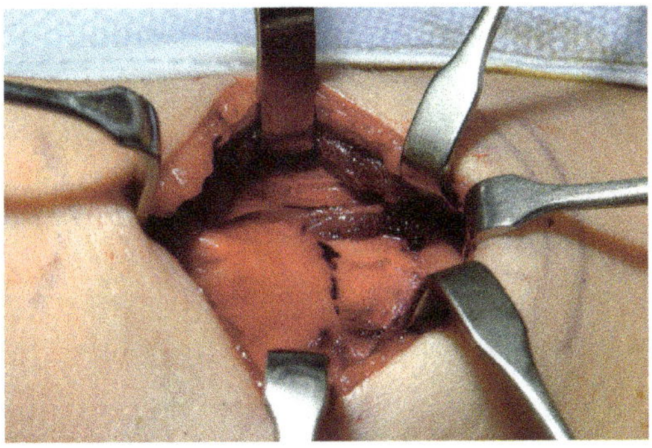

Figure 12.2: Passing the needle through the cricoid. Author image.

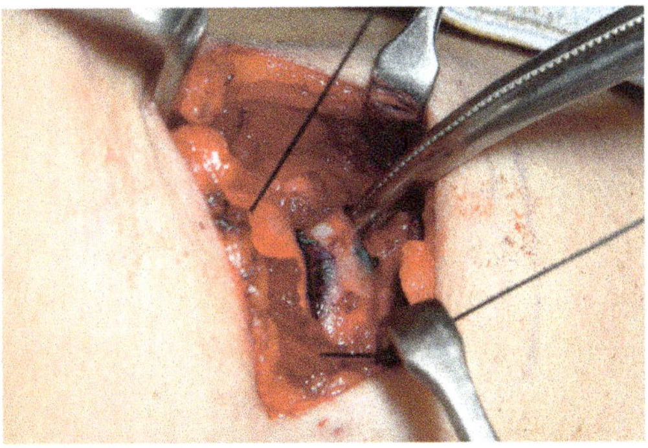

Figure 12.3: Approximation of cricoid and thyroid cartilage. Author image.

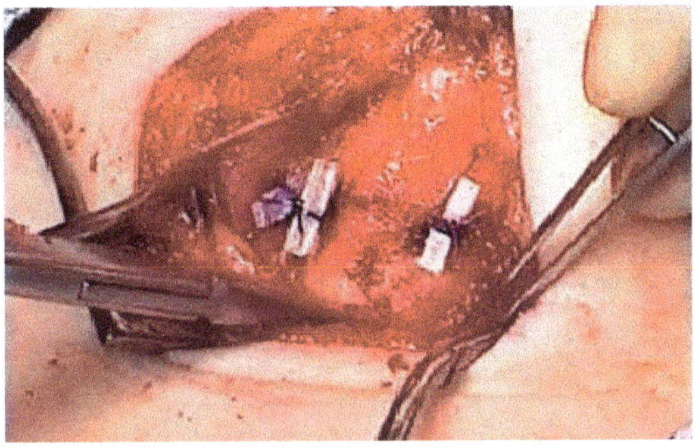

Figure 12.4: Bolsters in place: note the now smaller gap between the cricoid and thyroid cartilage. Author image.

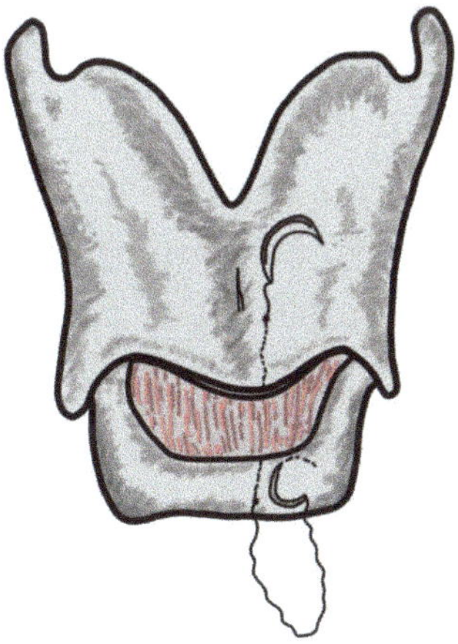

Figure 12.5: Schematic diagram of the positioning of sutures. Author image.

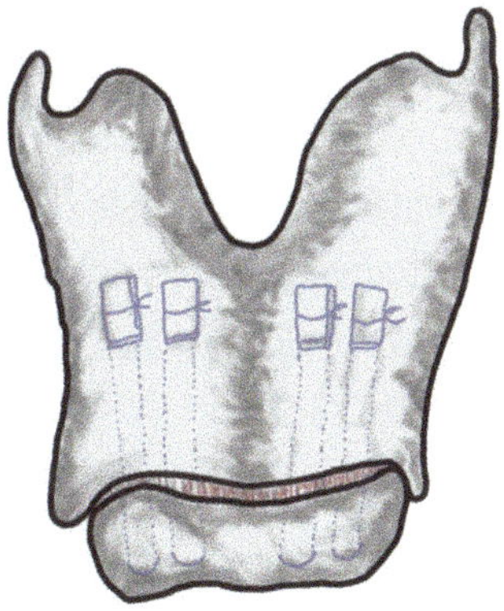

Figure 12.6: Schematic diagram of apposition from finished procedure: note the reduced cricothyroid distance. Author image.

are rarely required as the effect of paralysis is subtle and will usually improve with speech therapy.

Results of transgender surgery are variable. Surgical treatment of a mass-induced low pitch (which is essentially a thicker male vocal fold) by increasing the tension is limited – a thick rubber band will not produce a very high pitch no matter how far it is stretched. As a result, many surgeons have now moved away from CA and are performing endoscopic laryngeal surgery to reduce the mass and length of the folds. The pitch of the voice is raised, but the dynamic range of the voice may be narrowed. This is an important point to make the patient aware of before surgery as many find this restrictive, especially with the increased inflections of the female voice.

There are published results on the voice quality after CA and these have both quantitative and subjective results that are very good. We put more emphasis on the subjective scores as, ultimately, this is what shows patient satisfaction, and is the goal of surgery.

Pitch-increasing surgery has traditionally been limited to the CA procedure, although other surgical approaches have been advocated, including:

The 'laser assisted voice adjustment' results in an elevation of the fundamental frequency, but a diminution in the quality.

Vocal fold shortening procedures by deliberate creation of an anterior glottic web were described by Wendler. Pitch elevation is achieved; however, this comes at the cost of vocal quality, with a significant rise in the GRBAS score.

Feminization laryngoplasty involves removing the anterior portion of the thyroid cartilage and entering the airway; the vocal folds themselves are then tensioned, and around one third of the true vocal folds are excised. The anterior commissure is then recreated by suturing the anterior vocal folds together and then plating the anterior thyroid cartilage. This is a complex technique that appears to have quite variable results and (in the initial learning curve) may require revision operations. Patients who suffer complications typically have poor voice outcomes.

However, voice quality is not only dependent on fundamental frequency but also on the formants of the voice and other parameters such as breathiness, resonance, and prosody and there is an argument that even when successful in raising the pitch of the voice, this merely sounds like a falsetto male voice. Specialized centres where there is great experience in transgender patients include speech therapists which, in our opinion, can do more than CA to give the voice a female pattern and quality.

Summary

Cricothyroid approximation is a useful procedure in patients transitioning from male-to-female (transgender). Patient selection is important, and surgery should proceed only after careful evaluation by the multidisciplinary gender team. It is frequently the case that feminization of the voice (which comprises not only pitch, but also inflection and consonant production) can be achieved without the need for CA surgery. Other surgical techniques to increase vocal pitch have been described, but many of them appear to result in a deleterious effect on voice quality.

Further reading

Dacakis G, Oates J, Douglas J. 2012. Beyond voice: perception of gender in male-female transsexuals. *Curr Opinion Otolaryngol Head Neck Surgery* **20**(3):165–70.

Friedrich G, De Jong F, Mahieu H, et al. 2001. Laryngeal Framework Surgery: a proposal for classification and nomenclature by the Phonosurgery Committee of the European Laryngological Society. *Eur Arch Otorhinolaryngol* **258**(8):389–96.

Gibbins N, Bray D, Harries M. 2001. Long term quantitative results of an Isshiki Type IV thyroplasty: a case study. *J Voice* **25**(3):283–7.

Hong K, Ye M, Kim Y, Keovorkian K, et al. 1998. Functional differences between the two bellies of the cricothyroid muscle. *Otolaryngol Head Neck Surg* **118**(5):714–22.

Isshiki N, Morita H, Okamura H, Hiramoto M. 1974. Thyroplasty as a new phonosurgical technique. *Acta Otolaryngol* 78(5–6):726–31

Kanagalingam J, Georgalas C, Wood G, et al. 2005. Cricothyroid approximation and subluxation in 21 male to female transsexuals. *Laryngoscope* **115**(4):611–8.

Matal V, Cheesman A, Clarke P. 2003. Cricothyroid approximation and thyroid chondroplasty: a patient survey. *Otolaryngol Head Neck Surg* **126**(6):841–7.

Mu L, Sanders I. 2009. The human cricothyroid muscle: three muscle bellies and their innervation patterns. *J Voice* **23**(1):21–8.

Orestes M, Chhetri D. 2014. Superior laryngeal nerve injury, effects, clinical findings, prognosis and management options. *Curr Opinion Otolaryngol Head Neck Surg* **22**(6):439–43.

Orloff LA, Mann AP, Damrose JF, Goldman SN. 2006. Laser-assisted voice adjustment (LAVA) in transsexuals. *Laryngoscope* **116**:655–60.

Thomas JP, Macmillan C. 2013. Feminization laryngoplasty: assessment of surgical pitch elevation. *Eur Arch Otorhinolaryngol* **270**(10):2695–700.

Wendler J. 1990. Vocal pitch elevation after transexualism male to female. In: *Proceedings of the Union of the European Phoniatricians*. Salsomaggiore, Italy, UEP.

13

Laryngeal resizing for feminization of voice

James P. Thomas

Introduction

Once exposed to testosterone, typically during puberty, the thyroid cartilage enlarges, both increasing the internal luminal size of the larynx as well as altering the neck profile by visible protrusion of the Adam's apple. The vocal folds elongate and thicken, lowering the comfortable speaking pitch and lowest vocal pitch. There is usually a reduction of the upper vocal range and a change in the quality of the upper vocal range since thicker vocal folds must be stretched tighter to produce the same pitch as thinner vocal folds. The relaxed laryngeal position drops lower in the neck, increasing the internal length of the pharyngeal chamber, a longer chamber selectively amplifying the lower notes.

In individuals identifying as female gender (whether genetically male, intersex, or female), speech therapy or self-practice may result in learning to produce a desirable speaking vocal pitch and resonance, masking these changes induced by testosterone. These techniques utilize active muscle contraction of intrinsic laryngeal, pharyngeal, and cervical muscles, and require ongoing effort. Some individuals are successful in developing a habitual contraction, to the point of requiring conscious effort to lower their larynx into a typical genetic anatomic position and speak with their 'male voice'. However, most individuals note vocal fatigue or a neck ache from these attempts at maintaining female pitch and resonance through tonic muscle contraction. Even when successful, some individuals remain fearful of letting their guard down for even a moment in a sensitive situation where a masculine voice would be inappropriate. Some individuals are unable to accomplish any consistent change in pitch. As an ideal, after gender transition, comfortable speech would occur at a feminine pitch and with a feminine quality without having to think about contracting several muscles before every phonation. So either the individual acquires a female voice through practice until it becomes second nature, they live with a male voice, or they consider surgical modification of their phonatory tract.

Fundamental frequency of speech is one distinctive parameter in determination of a male versus female voice. A proposed fundamental frequency range for adult females is 145–275 Hz (D3–C♯4) and for males is 80–165 Hz (D♯2–E3). This leaves an area of overlap from 145–165 Hz (D3–E3) where fundamental frequency alone is not sufficient to determine the sex of a speaker. This is important as transgender patients with F0 as high as 181 Hz have been perceived as male. It appears that it is the interaction between F0, F0 range, intonation, and resonance that ultimately determines the perception of the speaker as female Addressing these components of speech as complements to each other would represent a more desirable approach to voice modification compared to fundamental pitch change alone.

Resonant frequency affects the gender perception of voice. This is especially true in the gray area where normal male and female speaking pitches overlap. The resonant frequency is inversely related to the length of the resonant tube, the pharynx. Speech therapy techniques have been used to modify the mouth opening and tongue placement. Günzburger noted that when comparing transexuals' male vs. female voices the resonance patterns change. Günzburger and others hypothesize that this is accomplished by practised manipulation of oropharyngeal shape and the elevation of the larynx. Elevation of the larynx enables higher resonant frequency of the pharynx, as the length of the resonant tube is decreased.

A number of pitch-altering surgeries have been pursued to address this frustration, including cricothyroid approximation (CTA), laser reduction vocal fold mass, anterior commissure advancement, and vocal fold webbing. None of these surgeries alter the size of the larynx, which has changed after exposure to testosterone.

CTA is one of the most common surgeries currently used to change the comfortable speaking pitch of the voice. The normal action of the cricothyroid muscle is to lengthen the vocal fold. The vocal quality produced by this increase in tension (via lengthening) of the vocal fold is called falsetto. Bringing the thyroid cartilage and cricoid cartilage into approximation in the anterior midline, CTA surgery sutures the cricothyroid muscle into a permanent position of contraction, although the degree is variable and the pitch elevation may range from an extreme falsetto to a mild falsetto quality of their voice. Some of my patients have described the perceived vocal quality as 'homosexual male', perhaps because tightening the cricothyroid muscle is a common approach genetic males utilize for raising comfortable speaking pitch.

Laser reduction of the vocal folds attempts to increase vocal pitch through a thinning and tightening of the vocal folds. Increases in fundamental frequency with this technique tend not to be as large as with other surgical methods. I have found, using an office KTP laser treatment, that a 1 to 2 semitone elevation has been the limit of pitch gain. Again, there is no change in the structure of the larynx.

Anterior commissure advancement was an early approach, which increases the protrusion of the thyroid cartilage, creating a more prominent Adam's apple. I am not aware of its continued use.

Webbing of the anterior portion of the vocal folds is a surgery designed to raise the comfortable speaking pitch by shortening the vibrating length of the vocal cords. It may also remove some of the lower pitches. Vocal fold mucosa is removed from the anterior true vocal fold's margins with scissors or laser and the anterior thyroarytenoid muscles are sewn together. It preserves the cricothyroid muscle so that an individual may still raise their pitch up into falsetto.

Significant laryngeal resizing began with Somyos Kunachak who proposed an open laryngoplasty to alter pitch. This procedure reduced the size of the larynx to a more female size in its cross-sectional dimension and shortened the length of the vibratory vocal fold. It possibly tensioned the vocal fold. It preserved the use of the cricothyroid muscle. Perhaps it thinned the vocal folds. Based primarily on this article, I began to perform what developed into a procedure termed feminization laryngoplasty or, as my first patient called it, 'FemLar'.

In transgender patients who were particularly adept at creating a female voice quality, I noted an ability to maintain, with muscle tension, two pharyngeal parameters: elevation of the larynx and narrowing of the pharynx. Based on a personal communication with Robert Bastian discussing this idea, I began to suspend the larynx higher in the neck (thyrohyoid elevation component). This might address one of the parameters, length of the pharyngeal chamber, leaving the patient to address the diameter of the chamber with muscle contraction if possible. This has become a standard part of the feminization laryngoplasty procedure.

I have also tried to reduce the diameter of the pharyngeal chamber in one patient, but I have not worked out a reliable technique to accomplish narrowing. Perhaps I removed an insufficient amount of tissue.

In summary, there are four procedures currently being used for modifying the genetic male voice an individual who identifies with the female gender. Cricothyroid approximation, web glottoplasty, laser thinning, and feminization laryngoplasty. Each of them alters the larynx anatomically in a different way.

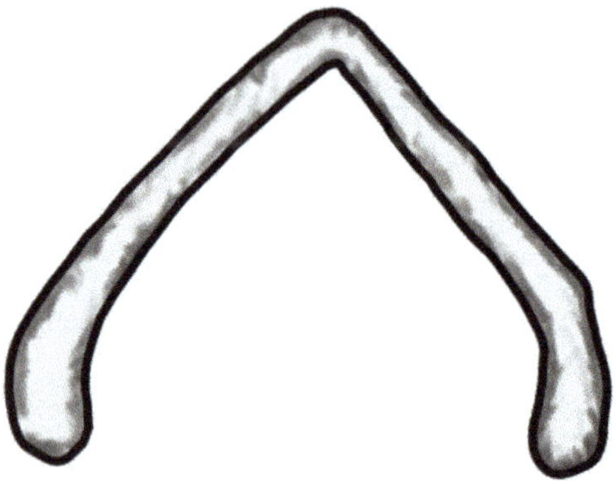

Figure 13.1: Coronal section of thyroid cartilage. Author image.

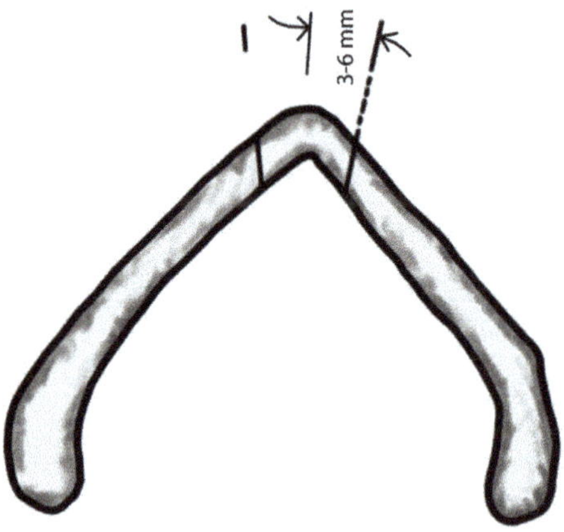

Figure 13.2: Coronal section of saw cuts. Author image.

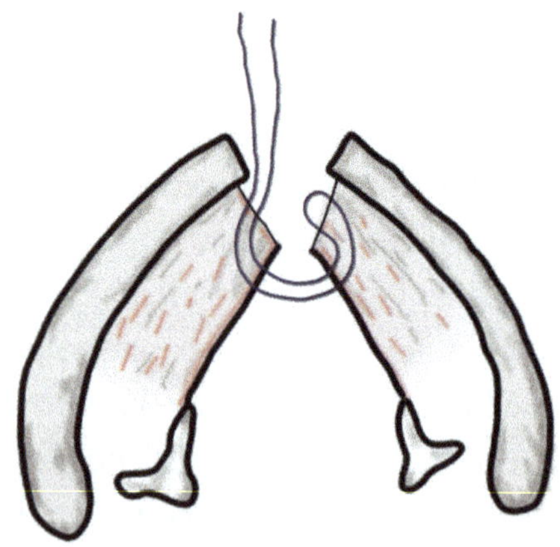

Figure 13.3: Coronal section – first CV-5 Gore-Tex horizontal mattress sutures. Author image. Path of stitch: (1) enters left TA muscle; (2) left vocal ligament; (3) left mucosa; (4) right mucosa; (5) right vocal ligament; (6) exits right TA muscle. Then is returned via the same path.

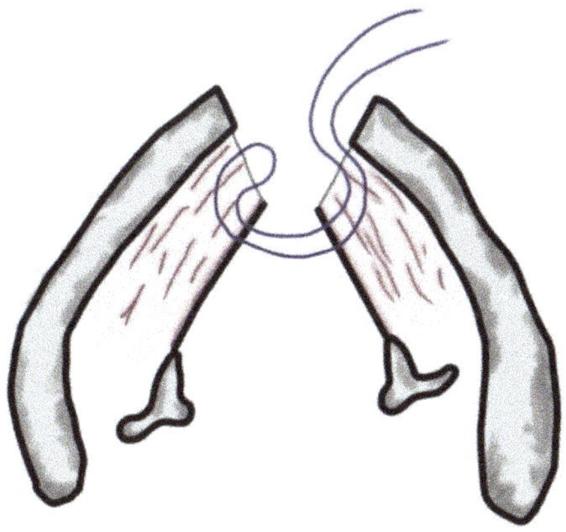

Figure 13.4: Coronal section – second CV-5 Gore-Tex horizontal mattress sutures. Author image.

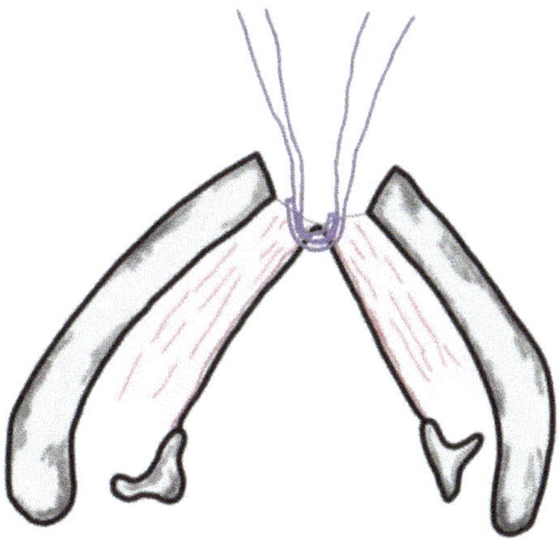

Figure 13.5: Coronal section – both Gore-Tex sutures pulling anteriorly in true folds to create anterior commissure. Author image.

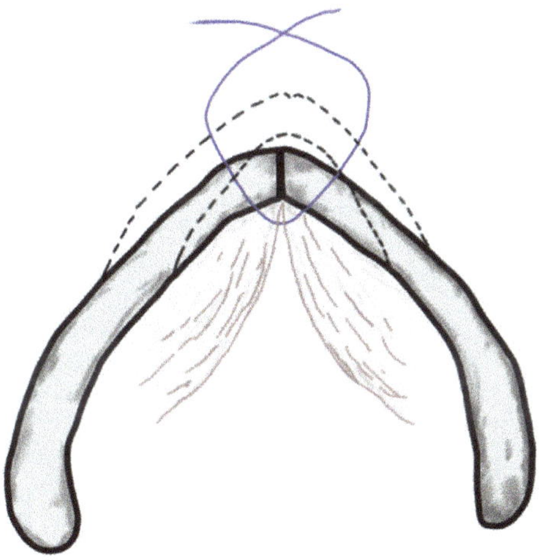

Figure 13.6: Coronal section – after closure. Author image.

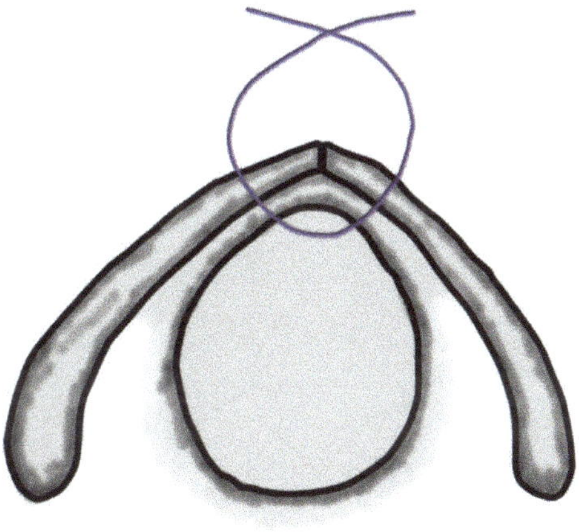

Figure 13.7: Coronal section – after closure at the level of subglottis. Author image.

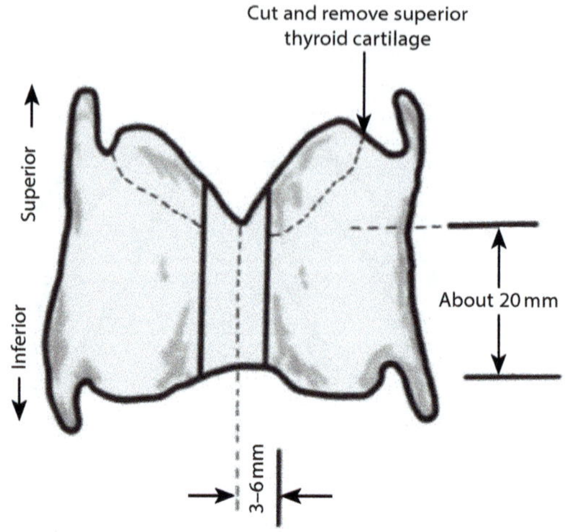

Figure 13.8: Anterior view. Author image.

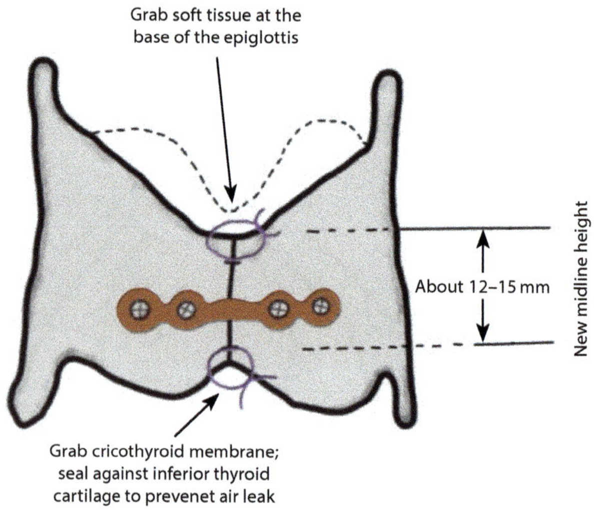

Figure 13.9: Anterior closed view. Author image.

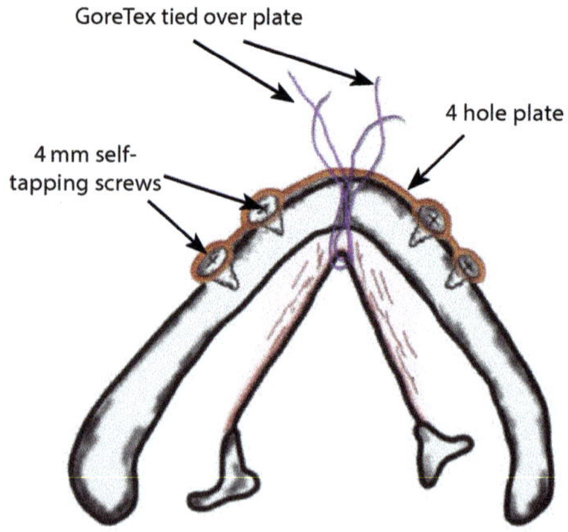

Figure 13.10: Coronal closed view. Author image.

Feminization laryngoplasty – procedure

Anesthesia

The procedure is performed under general endotracheal anesthesia using a 6-0 endotracheal tube.

Antibiotics

Clindamycin and cefotaxime are administered at the time of surgery. Seven days of post-operative oral therapy with either cefuroxime or levofloxacin is also given. Typically the intravenous administration of antibiotics is completed before the time of surgical entry into the airway. The wound is irrigated with normal saline containing 100,000 units per litre of bacitracin prior to closure.

Steroids

At the beginning of surgery, 10 mg of dexamethasone is given intravenously. Oral prednisone or methylprednisolone are given post-operatively in selected cases if significant swelling develops one to three days later.

Technique

Note that all photos are taken from the perspective of the anaesthetist at the head of the table.

Step 1

- Approximately 5 cm incision placed in or parallel to a skin crease directly in the midline.
- Strap muscles are separated in the midline exposing anatomy from the hyoid bone to the upper cricothyroid membrane.
- See Figure 13.11.

Step 2

- Marks are placed 5–7 mm lateral to the midline on each side of the thyroid cartilage.
- The upper 10 mm of the thyroid cartilage alae are marked for removal.
- The upper portions of the thyroid cartilage are removed.
- The thyroid cartilage is divided vertically with an oscillating saw about 4–7 mm on either side of midline with the saw kerf removing about one additional millimeter of cartilage. The goal is to narrow the internal aper-

ture of the laryngeal glottis by collapsing the thyroid alae medially. A prior cricothyroid approximation may preclude this removal.

- Cuts placed at a 90° angle to the cartilage allow only the inner thyroid lamina to approximate. The inner lamina is more contoured than the outer lamina with an internal bulge inferior to the vocal folds. A 90° cut thus prevents an airtight closure unless these contours are then removed with a cutting burr.

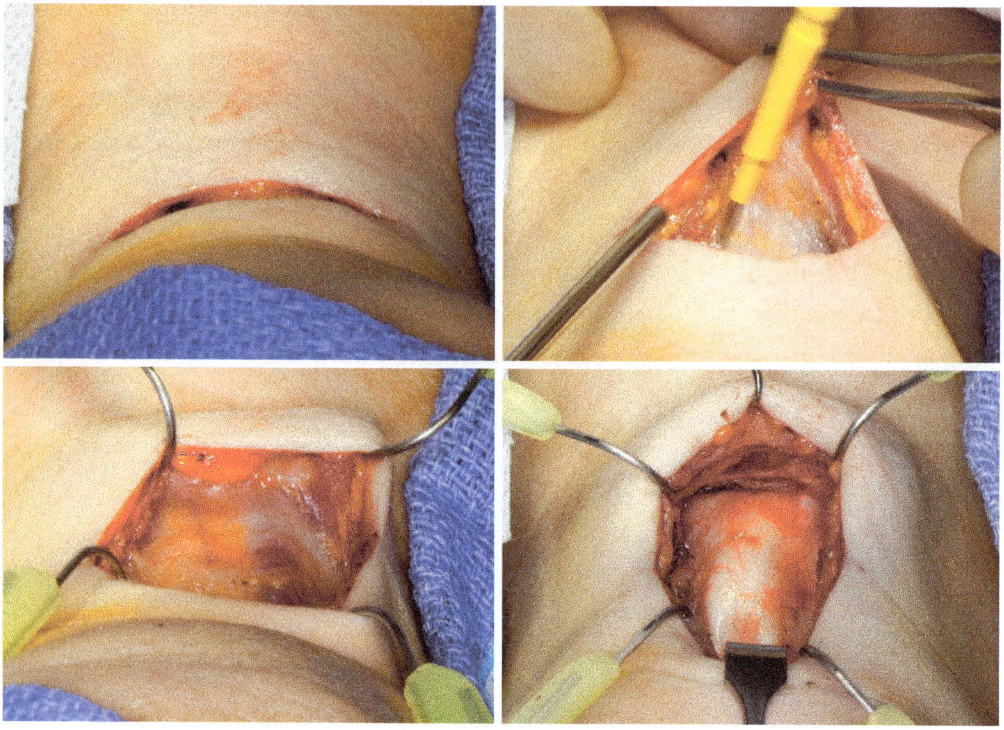

Figure 13.11: Incision, dissection, retraction, and exposure. Image courtesy of Thomas.

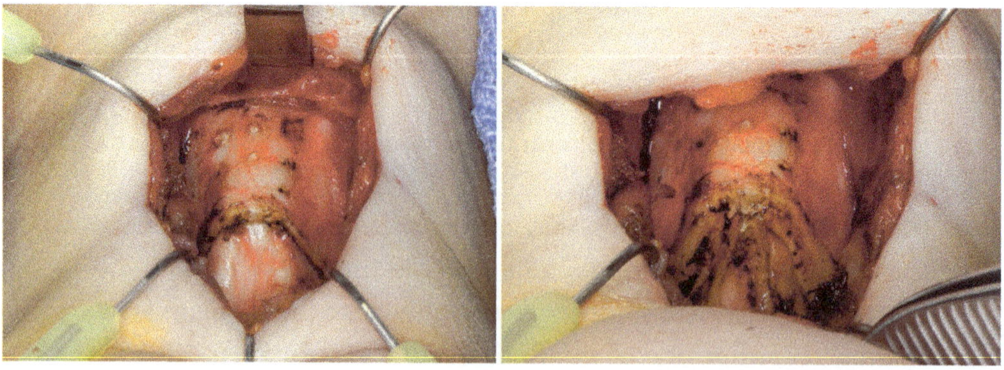

Figure 13.12: Marking on the thyroid cartilage. Image courtesy of Thomas.

- Direct sagittal cuts allow only the outer lamina to approximate when the alae are collapsed back into the midline.
- Beveling the cuts between these two planes allows complete, airtight closure of the new anterior larynx in the midline. If tight closure is precluded by an inappropriate saw angle or because of any variation of thickness in the cartilage, adjust with a cutting burr.
- See Figure 13.12.

Step 3

- The central strip of anterior thyroid cartilage is elevated away from inner soft tissue and removed with electrocautery.
- Removal of the vertical anterior thyroid cartilage segment will both narrow the internal laryngeal aperture and very effectively remove the Adam's apple contour (more completely than a 'tracheal shave'). The airway is not typically entered though, if it is, penetration usually occurs in the thinnest area, which is just superior to the anterior commissure.
- See Figure 13.13.

Step 4

- The thyroid alae may be retracted laterally for a better view of the internal glottis. The vocal fold anterior ligaments are identified.
- The airway is incised just superior to the anterior commissure. Split the false vocal folds.
- See Figure 13.14.

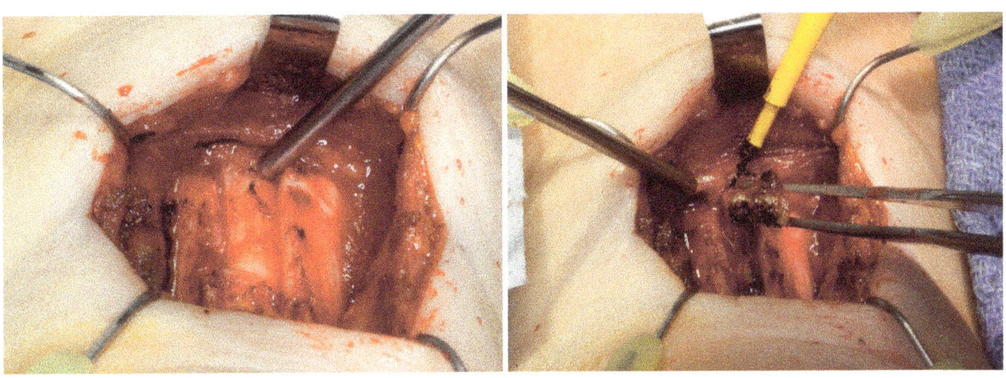

Figure 13.13: Removal of the vertical anterior thyroid cartilage segment. Image courtesy of Thomas.

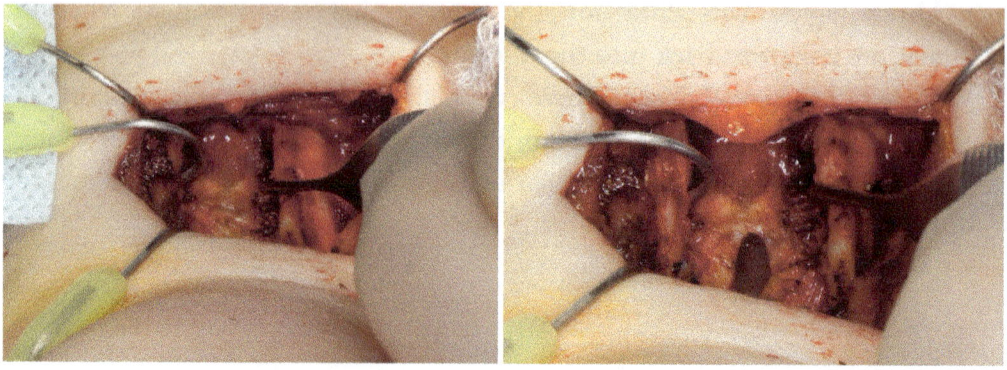

Figure 13.14: Retraction of thyroid alae to view internal glottis and incision superior to the anterior commissure. Image courtesy of Thomas.

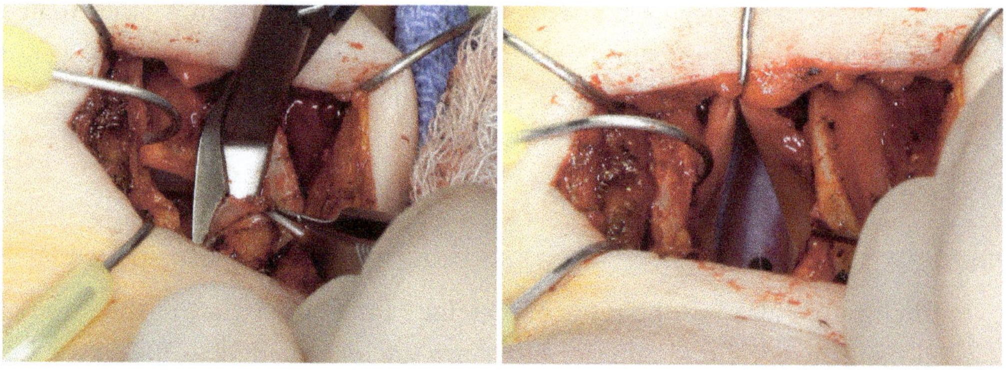

Figure 13.15: Modification of the anterior third of both false folds and assessment of the anterior glottic ligament to confirm the amount of tension on the vocal folds. Image courtesy of Thomas.

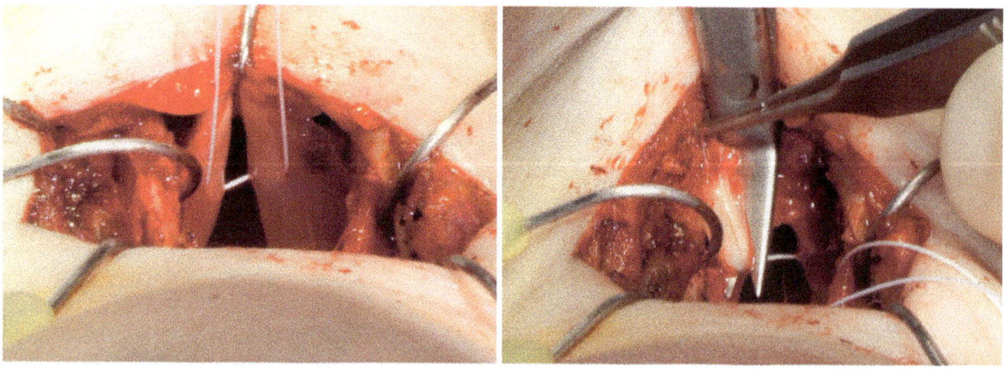

Figure 13.16: Use of a Gore-Tex suture to mark the membranous vocal folds for removal. Image courtesy of Thomas.

Step 5

- Approximately the anterior third of each false vocal fold is removed, likely including the saccule reducing the diameter of the supraglottis after surgery. During surgery, this also provides an improved view of the true vocal folds and more space to manipulate needles within the larynx.
- Pull on the anterior glottic ligament assessing how much of the anterior vocal folds need to be removed in order to collapse the thyroid alae back into the midline while maintaining tension on the vocal folds.
- See Figure 13.15.

Step 6

- Using half of a double-ended 4-0 polytetrafluroethylene (Gore-Tex) suture mark the membranous vocal folds for removal.
- Include the vocal ligament in this suture to maintain not only a symmetric length to the neo-vocal folds, but also to maintain the vibratory margin's vertical symmetry.
- Remove the membranous vocal fold and thyroarytenoid muscle anterior to the marking suture.
- Minimize the length of the incision inferior to the vocal folds keeping the inferior extent of the excision beneath the lower boundary of the thyroid cartilage. If the subglottic incision continues beyond the inferior edge of the thyroid cartilage into the cricothyroid membrane, it is more difficult to obtain an airtight closure.
- See Figure 13.16.

Step 7

- The vocal folds are stretched as the thyroid lamina are brought back together to verify they are not too long to be placed under tension when secured against the remaining inner thyroid lamina. If they will not be under adequate tension, more vocal fold can be removed.
- Using Gore-Tex, a horizontal mattress suture is placed. The needle enters the left thyroarytenoid muscle, passes through the vocal ligament (which feels slightly dense) and includes about 1 mm of medial margin vocal fold epithelium. Exit at the upper vibratory lip of the membranous vocal fold. This passes into the opposite fold at a corresponding location beginning with the vocal fold epithelium and passing out through the thyroarytenoid

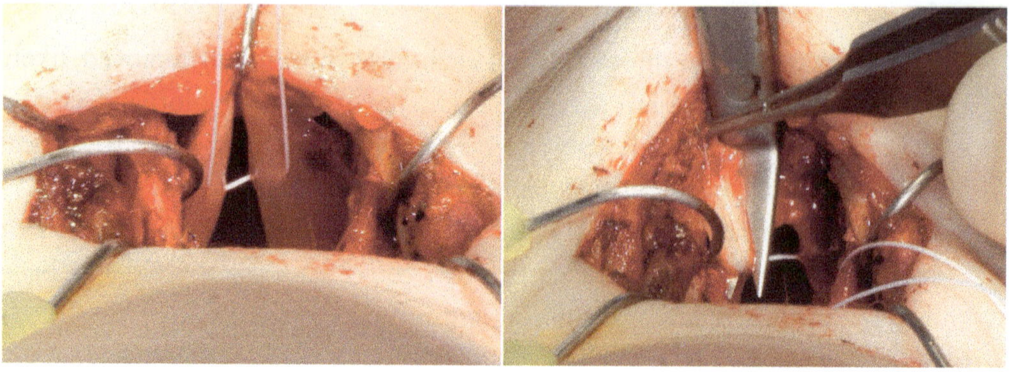

Figure 13.17: Securing the vocal ligaments. Image courtesy of Thomas.

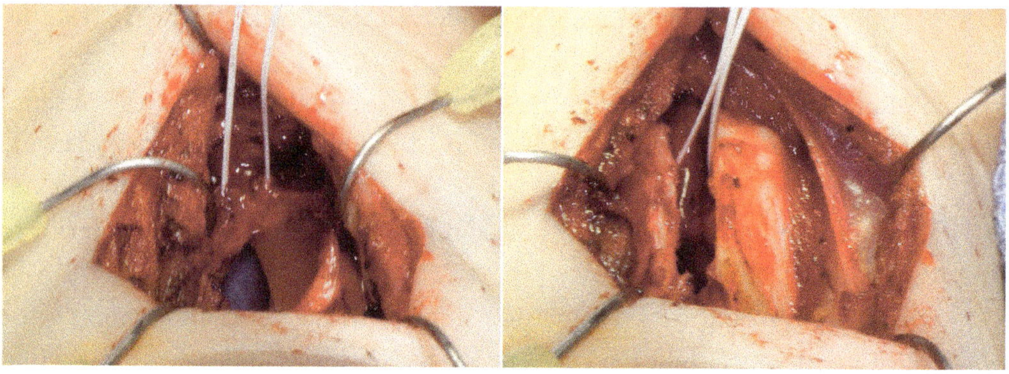

Figure 13.18: Using the Gore-Tex marking suture to oppose the new anterior commissure. Image courtesy of Thomas.

muscle. I re-pass the needle back following a path about 1 mm inferior at the new inferior vibratory lip of the membranous vocal fold. Both ends of this first suture exit the left thyroarytenoid muscle.

- See Figure 13.17.

Step 8

- Remove the Gore-Tex marking suture, reusing it, passing it in opposition using a similar pattern beginning with the right thyroarytenoid muscle. At the conclusion, both ends of one suture exit the left vocal fold and both ends of the other suture exit the right vocal fold. Pulling on these brings the new anterior commissure together.

- When the thyroid alae are brought back together, the slipperiness of the Gore-Tex allows it to slide between the cartilage halves.
- See Figure 13.18.

Step 9 – Hyoid

- Muscles are elevated from the anterior, inferior half of the hyoid bone with electrocautery.
- Strap muscles are divided at their insertion along the inferior edge of the hyoid bone for 15 mm either side of midline.

Step 10 – Drilling

- 1 mm holes are drilled in the new anterior edge of each thyroid cartilage, one inferior at the level of the subglottis, and one superior at the level of the false vocal folds.
- Each hole is angled toward the midline internally.
- Two additional holes are placed along each superior border of the thyroid cartilage where the upper wings were removed. The softer the cartilage, the further from the upper cut edge of thyroid cartilage; I place these holes to avoid tear-out later when tightening.
- Four holes are drilled into the hyoid bone, two either side of midline. These are angled slightly inferiorly to allow passage of the large needle.

Step 11 – Closure

- Four braided, non-absorbable sutures are individually passed through each hole in the superior edge of the thyroid cartilage and then through a corresponding hole in the hyoid bone. No sutures are tied yet.
- A 4-0 monofilament suture (nylon or poliglecaprone (Monocryl)) is placed through the upper holes in the superior thyroid cartilage and internally includes the cut edges of the false vocal folds with the intent of pulling them against the inner thyroid lamina during closure. Leave this needle attached temporarily.
- A 4-0 suture is passed through the inferior holes and includes the cut edge of the subglottic mucosa, again with the intent that the mucosa will reattach to the inner thyroid perichondrium and that there will be an airtight seal in the immediate post-operative period. Leave this needle attached temporarily.

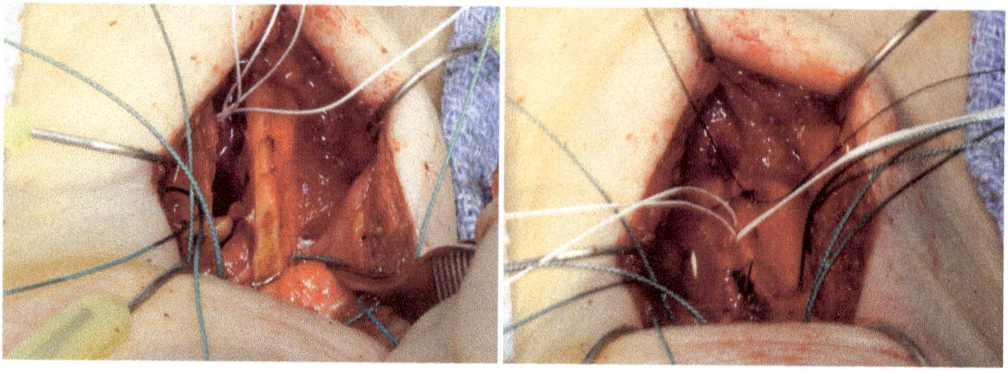

Figure 13.19: Closure with sutures. Image courtesy of Thomas.

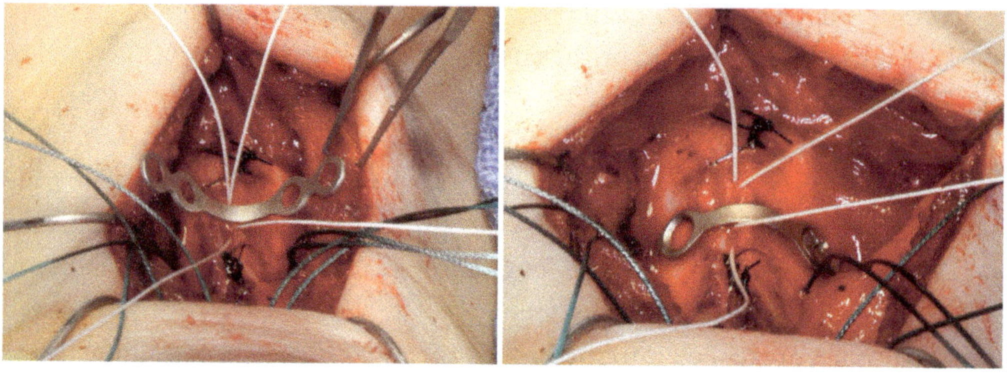

Figure 13.20: Assessment of closure with plate. Image courtesy of Thomas.

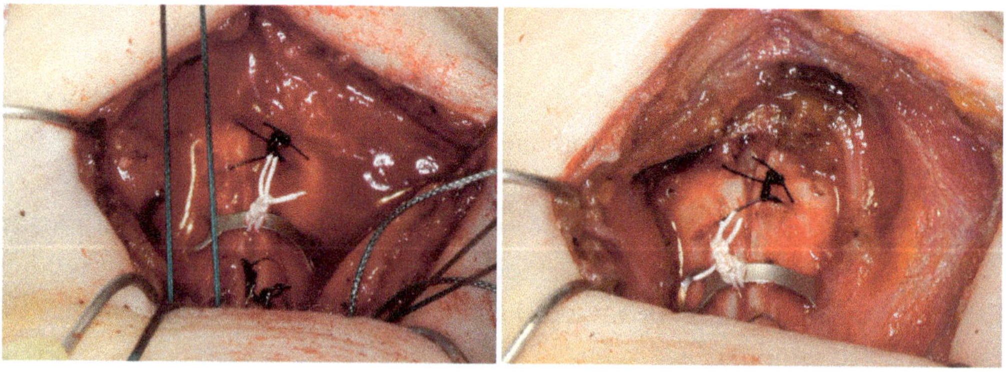

Figure 13.21: Tightening of sutures and preparation for wound closure. Image courtesy of Thomas.

- Bring the edges of the thyroid cartilage together and suture closed.
- With the needle still on the upper suture, tissue at the base of the epiglottis is pulled tight against the upper border of the thyroid cartilage.
- The inferior needle pulls the soft tissue of the cricothyroid membrane against the inferior border.
- See Figure 13.19.

Step 12

- A 4-hole, dogbone shaped plate is bent to the shape of the newly angled anterior thyroid cartilage. It is placed preferably at the same level as the original attachment of the anterior commissure. 4 mm, self-tapping screws are placed bilaterally.
- The Gore-Tex suture slides between the coopted edges of the thyroid cartilage, tightened and tied around the plate to maintain the new anterior commissure against the inner thyroid perichondrium.
- See Figure 13.20.

Step 13

- The 0-Ethibond sutures are then tightened and tied, pulling the larynx superiorly in the neck. Typically the thyroid cartilage does not quite reach the hyoid bone.
- The wound is irrigated with saline solution containing Bacitracin. The strap muscles are re-approximated and can be slightly plicated, pulled superiorly and reattached to the hyoid bone under some tension. Subcutaneous tissues are closed with 4-0 Monocryl.
- The skin is closed with a running subcuticular suture, either 4-0 Monocryl. I place some form of cyanoacrylate on the skin.
- A nasogastric tube is passed momentarily into the stomach and the contents aspirated. The patient is extubated and awakened.
- See Figure 13.21.

Post-operative

- Surgery is performed as a daycase.
- Each patient is discharged after approximately one hour into the care of a friend, family or a professional caregiver for the first 24 hours post-operatively.

- Flexible laryngoscopy is performed every day for three days.
- Monitor for:
  - subcutaneous emphysema;
  - supraglottic edema; and
  - neck swelling or erythema.
- Instructions:
  - Two weeks of complete voice rest are suggested.
  - Pain is typically fairly minimal (though individually variable). A narcotic is prescribed for use against pain and for cough suppression.
  - Nothing heavier than ten pounds is to be lifted for one month. Other forms of straining, such as Valsalva maneouvre, are strongly discouraged.
  - No elective endotracheal intubations for three months. If intubated for general anesthesia, she should request a number 6 endotracheal tube be used.

Caveats and thoughts

Prior CTA surgery: after CTA surgery, the cricoid and thyroid cartilage are typically fused. Even if they can be pried or sawed apart, the cricothyroid joint is non-functional. Utilize a midline thyrotomy division and do not remove any additional central thyroid cartilage. The cricothyroid fusion limits opening of the thyroid cartilage and surgical exposure. With a prior CTA, the post-operative FemLar patient has only a shortened thyroarytenoid muscle for pitch alteration, but no cricothyroid muscle for additional upper vocal range.

Post-operative airway compromise: obstructive oedema may occur on the posterior aspect of the arytenoids from two probable aetiologies. One is infectious. The other seems to be from extension of the resection along the superior edge of the thyroid cartilage toward the superior thyroid cornu.

Oedema seems to peak on post-operative day number three. Infections seem to be identifiable by day three or else an infection tends not to occur.

A temporary tracheostomy and drainage may be required for an infection.

If an infection occurs, the plate, GoreTex and Ethibond sutures will likely need to be removed. If removed after one month, they are no longer needed and the anterior commissure remains well attached.

Risks and treatments

- A KTP laser may tighten the superior vocal cord surface correcting asymmetric tension.
- The laser can also be applied bilaterally to raise the pitch further.
- Most patients note a loss of volume, both in everyday speech and for a yell. In most cases she cannot replicate the volume of her previous voice. Subjectively, some patients are pleased with the softness of their new voice or may consider it a reasonable trade-off.
- Numerous patients do not initially perceive a change in their voice after surgery. While documentation is important in many respects (for the surgeon to learn what works, legal documentation, etc.), it is invaluable to the patient as well, in order to hear the difference in voice after treatment. After hearing the pre and post-operative recordings, many patients gain confidence in their new female voice.

Conclusion

Feminization laryngoplasty, including a thyrohyoid elevation component and possibly a later post-operative laser tuning, is a surgical approach designed for individuals wishing to transition from a male to female gender voice by increasing the fundamental and possibly the resonant frequencies of her voice.

Further reading

Brown M, et al. 2000. Pitch change in male-to-female transsexuals: has phonosurgery a role to play? *Int J Lang Comm Dis* **35**(1):129–36.

Carew L, Dacakis G, Oates J. 2007. The effectiveness of oral resonance therapy on the perception of femininity of voice in male-to-female transsexuals. *J Voice* **21**(5):591–603.

Dacakis G. 2000. Long-term maintenance of fundamental frequency increases in male-to-female transsexuals. *J Voice* **14**(4):549–56.

Donald PJ. 1982. Voice change surgery in the transsexual. *Head Neck Surg* **4**(5):433–7.

Gross M. 1999. Pitch-raising surgery in male-to-female transsexuals. *J Voice* **13**(2):5.

Günzburger D. 1989. Voice adaptation by transsexuals. *Clin Linguist Phonet* **3**:10.

Hong KH, et al. 1998. Functional differences between the two bellies of the cricothyroid muscle. *Otolaryngol Head Neck Surg* **118**(5):9.

Isshiki N, Morita H, Okamura H, Hiramoto M. 1974. Thyroplasty as a new phonosurgical technique. *Acta Otolaryng* **78**(1):8.

Isshiki N, Taira T, Tanabe M. 1983. Surgical alteration of the vocal pitch. *J Otolaryngol* **12**(5):6.

Isshiki N. 1998. Mechanical and dynamic aspects of voice production as related to voice therapy and phonosurgery. *J Voice* **12**(2):13.

Kocak I, Akpınar ME, Cakır ZA, et al. 2010. Laser reduction glottoplasty for managing androphonia after failed cricothyroid approximation surgery. *J Voice* **24**(6):758–64.

Kunachak S, Prakunhungsit S, Sujjalak K. 2000. Thyroid cartilage and vocal fold reduction: a new phonosurgical method for male-to-female transsexuals. *Ann Otol Rhinol Laryngol* **109**:5.

Matai V, Cheesman AD, Clarke PM. 2003. Cricothyroid approximation and thyroid chondroplasty: a patient survey. *Otolaryngol Head Neck Surg* **128**(6):841–7.

Neumann K. Welzel C. 2004. The importance of the voice in male-to-female transsexualism. *J Voice* **18**(1):153–67.

Orloff LA, Mann AP, Damrose JF, Goldman SN. 2006. Laser-assisted voice adjustment (LAVA) in transsexuals. *Laryngoscope* **116**(4):655–60.

Remacle M, Matar N, Morsomme D, et al. 2011. Glottoplasty for male-to-female transsexualism: voice results. *J Voice* **25**(1):120–3.

Tucker HM. 1985. Anterior commissure laryngoplasty for adjustment of vocal fold tension. *Ann Otol Rhinol Laryngol* **94**(6 Pt 1):547–9.

Wagner I, Fugain C, Monneron-Girard L, et al. 2003. Pitch-raising surgery in fourteen male-to-female transsexuals. *Laryngoscope* **113**:9.

Wendler J. 1990. Vocal pitch elevation after transexualism male to female. In: *Proceedings of the Union of the European Phoniatricians*. Salsomaggiore, Italy: UEP.

Yang CY, Palmer AD, Murray KD, et al. 2002. Cricothyroid approximation to elevate vocal pitch in male-to-female transsexuals: results of surgery. *Ann Otol Rhinol Laryngol* **111**(6):477–85.

SECTION VI: PAEDIATRIC SURGERY

14

Vocal fold augmentation in children

Prasad Thottam and Deepak Mehta

Introduction

Vocal fold immobility (VFI) is a surprisingly common ailment in children, and identification is rising with increased awareness and diagnostic evaluations. Unlike the adult population, the most common cause of unilateral VFI in children is iatrogenic. With the increased prevalence of patent ductus arteriosus ligations being performed, associated left vocal fold paralysis/paresis accounts for the majority of these cases. Other iatrogenic causes cited are: intubation, tracheoesophageal fistula repair, spinal fusion, chiari decompression, branchial anomaly excision, and thyroidectomy. With the above in mind, idiopathic, anatomical, infectious, and malignant causes for VFI still do occur in this population.

Stridor has been reported in up to 70% of children presenting with unilateral VFI and is the most common presenting symptom. While, in surveys, dysphonia was cited as the most common presentation in children and adults, the neonatal population exhibits high rates of feeding difficulties and associated aspiration signs. These findings often require further investigation through flexible fibreoptic laryngoscopy (FFL) at a minimum.

Diagnosis

Once a patient presents with symptoms suggesting the possibility of an airway anomaly, if they are clinically stable, a FFL is the safest and easiest way to acquire maximal objective information. In the unilateral VFI patient this should ideally be recorded, in order to review in half or quarter speed, and if stroboscopy is available it should be utilized. This will allow a more thorough examination and is of particular importance when viewing time is limited. If VFI is demonstrated, then a direct laryngoscopy and bronchoscopy (DLB) may be indicated to determine the possible aetiology and also to examine for synchronous lesions. If a patient is intubated or not stable for FFL at bedside, the patient can be weaned from sedation, or placed in twilight and the VF mobility can be assessed prior to the DLB being performed.

Direct laryngoscopy and bronchoscopy is performed in the operating room and allows for an entire comprehensive examination of the airway. Synchronous airway lesions have been reported to be present in as many as 45% of patients with VFI. During this process, possible aetiology for VFI and other airway lesions can be investigated in a controlled environment. Under anaesthesia, the cricoarytenoid joint can be palpated for possible fixation and examined for anterior or posterior glottic webs that may limit mobility. It is only after these have been ruled out that the term vocal fold paralysis (VFP) can be accurately used.

If VFP is determined as the aetiology of immobility, laryngeal electromyography may play a role in the establishment of prognosis, but to date the data in paediatrics is limited. True VFP recovery has been reported to range from one month up to eleven years. It is for this reason that it is generally recommended that clinicians allow at least one year from diagnosis before any permanent thyroplasty or augmentation techniques are utilized in paediatric and adult clients alike.

Intervention

It has been estimated that in up to 80% of cases of unilateral VFI, effective contralateral VF compensation will occur without intervention. In those patients who do not adequately compensate further surgical treatment can be considered. It should always be remembered when discussing interventions with patients and families that they are informed that currently, no procedure can restore normal vocal fold motion and that these procedures assist only in improving glottic insufficiency. It is also in good practice to discuss how speech therapy may be beneficial pre- and post-surgical intervention. In select cases, older children with unilateral VFI have achieved improved glottic closure and voice quality through speech therapy.

Injection laryngoplasty

Also referred to as vocal fold augmentation, this procedure is the most common and most conservative surgical option for unilateral VFI associated glottic insufficiency. The materials commonly utilized for injection are temporary for a range of different timeframes and are biodegradable. This is often advantageous in the management of the paediatric patient, for whom the potential of a natural return to VF function is high, unless witnessed injury or neural disruption has occurred. This is especially true in cases involving young infants.

Rating of the different injectable materials in the paediatric population by both length of time of appropriate voice quality and effectiveness has been carried out in various studies. Calcium hydroxylapatite has been reported to maintain effectiveness for 12–24 months, while acellular dermis or collagen has demonstrated improvement for 4–6 months. For more short-term medialization, autologous fat has demonstrated improvement for up to 6 months and absorbable gelatin powder for 4–6 weeks. Regardless of material, data has demonstrated improvement of symptoms in patients. In one study, 94% of patients demonstrated improvement of hoarseness and 85% had dysphagia or aspiration improvement.

Thyroplasty

Permanent vocal fold augmentation and medialization techniques are generally viewed as a last resort in children, and only to be utilized when there is confirmed glottis incompetence and/or permanent neural paralysis. In these situations, the authors recommend the patient be clinically stable and have confirmatory imaging, laryngoscopy evaluation, and laryngeal EMG prior to procedure. There have been reports of permanent medialization procedures being performed before the age of two years, though we stress that this is only for the most exceptional of cases.

When performing thyroplasty techniques, certain paediatric attributes must be taken into account. The paediatric thyroid cartilage and laryngeal apparatus is smaller, more malleable, and the vocal folds are positioned lower. For children, passive respiration is more difficult as they are subject to further growth, both of which must be taken into account. Lastly, patient cooperation is highly unlikely so it is recommended that this procedure be performed under general anaesthesia via laryngeal mask anaesthesia or tracheostomy.

To date, studies examining thyroplasty in children have been limited to case report and case series information. In a particular study, Goretex ribbon (W. L. Gore & Associates, Flagstaff, Arizona) was the material utilized for medialization on three patients, one of whom developed aspiration pneumonia post-operatively. There is little data or information regarding the long term voice results or movement of the Gortex as the child grows or goes through puberty. Lastly, the data and reports are sparse when examining cricothyroid joint subluxation and adduction arytenoidopexy. The current view is that these procedures should be limited and used only for minor alterations/adjustments in post-pubescent teens that have undergone thyroplasty.

Laryngeal reinnervation

In recent years, the possibility and feasibility of recurrent laryngeal reinnervation has been explored and described. This is accomplished through performing a neurorraphy between the proximal end of the ansa-cervicalis nerve and the distal end of the recurrent laryngeal nerve (RLN). The goal of this procedure is to increase tone of the affected muscles – specifically, the thyroarytenoid and interarytenoid. In a very limited study examining this technique in children, improvements in tone, phonation time and glottic closure were demonstrated in the majority of patients. With the above in mind, we feel this is a possible option for known confirmed permanent RLN paralysis and may yield long-term benefit in certain individuals.

Table 14.1: Procedure and associated limitations.

Procedure	**Limitation**
Injection laryngoplasty	Temporary; risk of subglottic injection
Thyroplasty	Permanent; lack of data on effect on the growing larynx; >2 years of age before being considered; tracheotomy or LMA for procedure; graft extrusion
Reinnervation	External incision; only described in adolescents; improves voice and tone
Speech therapy	Requires patient cooperation and compensatory mechanisms

Conclusion

Vocal fold augmentation and thyroplasty remain the primary forms of treatment in paediatric unilateral VFI. While newer techniques such as laryngeal reinnervation demonstrate promise, there is little evidence in regard to risk/benefit analysis and effectiveness in the paediatric population. This primarily involves vocal projection, not aspiration risk. Overall, unilateral VFI often resolves or can be compensated for in the paediatric population; it is our practice to utilize temporizing injection laryngoplasty techniques and defer permanent thyroplasty until adolescence or other conservative options have been exhausted (Table 14.1).

Further reading

Cohen MS, Mehta DK, Maguire RC, Simons JP. 2011. Injection medialization laryngoplasty in children. *Arch Otolaryngol Head Neck Surg* **137**:264–8.

Daya H, Hosni A, Bejar-Solar I, et al. 2000. Pediatric vocal fold paralysis: a long-term retrospective study. *Arch Otolaryngol Head Neck Surg* **126**:21–5.

Ishman SL, Halum SL, Patel NJ, et al. 2006. Management of vocal paralysis: a comparison of adult and pediatric practices. *Otolaryngol Head Neck Surg* **135**:590–4.

King EF, Blumin JH. 2009. Vocal cord paralysis in children. *Curr Opin Otolaryngol Head Neck Surg* **17**:483–7.

Parikh SR. 2004. Pediatric unilateral vocal fold immobility. *Otolaryngologic Clinics of North America* **237**:203–15.

Rosin DF, Handler SD, Potsic WP, et al. 1990. Vocal cord paralysis in children. *Laryngoscope* **100**:1174–9.

Schindler A, Bottero A, Capaccio P, et al. 2008. Vocal improvement after voice therapy in unilateral vocal fold paralysis. *J Voice* **22**:113–8.

Scott AR, Chong PS, Hartnick CJ, Randolph GW. 2010. Spontaneous and evoked laryngeal electromyography of the thyroarytenoid muscles: a canine model for intraoperative recurrent laryngeal nerve monitoring. *Ann Otol Rhinol Laryngol* **119**:54–63.

Setlur J, Hartnick CJ. 2012. Management of unilateral true vocal cord paralysis in children. *Curr Opin Otolaryngol Head Neck Surg* **20**:497–501.

Sipp JA, Kerschner JE, Braune N, Hartnick CJ. 2007. Vocal fold medialization in children: injection laryngoplasty, thyroplasty, or nerve reinnervation? *Arch Otolaryngol Head Neck Surg* **133**:767–71.

Smith ME, Roy N, Stoddard K. 2008. Ansa-RLN reinnervation for unilateral vocal fold paralysis in adolescents and young adults. *Int J Pediatr Otorhinolaryngol* **72**:1311–6.

Truong MT, Messner AH, Kerschner JE, et al. 2007. Pediatric vocal fold paralysis after cardiac surgery: rate of recovery and sequelae. *Otolaryngol Head Neck Surg* **137**:780–4.

Zur KB. 2012. Recurrent laryngeal nerve reinnervation for unilateral vocal fold immobility in children. *Laryngoscope* **122**(Suppl 4):S82–3.

SECTION VII: DEVELOPING TECHNIQUES

15

Future techniques in phonosurgery

Markus Hess

Introduction

In a practical book such as this, the main aim is to inform and guide the phonosurgeon on 'how to . . .' perform phonosurgery and avoid problems and risks. The design of this book is therefore to offer support by sharing what is already known and what proved useful. However, as always in science and medicine, there may be insights that, at this point, are 'just ideas and thoughts', but may have the potential to grow and might induce a shift to other phonosurgical techniques in the future. It is with this in mind that the Editors have afforded the opportunity to contribute some ideas to this laryngeal framework guide – ideas 'out of the box' that came up in recent years during discussions with experienced surgeons, as well as creative newcomers at numerous meetings and courses on phonosurgery.

The ideas mentioned here certainly do not reflect the enormous creativity from phonosurgeons from all over the world. However, if there is one basic denominator of most ideas it might be the urge to simplify or refine surgical techniques and instrumentation so that more and more colleagues are motivated to perform such operations. It is the aim of this brief chapter to introduce some thoughts and ideas so that readers may further develop the techniques presented in this book, or come up with their own modifications. Or even better, invent new ideas to refine phonosurgical treatment for our patients.

Potentially helpful techniques for phonosurgical interventions

Digital volume tomography in the planning of thyroplasty implants

Rationale

Digital volume tomography (DVT) allows for three dimensional and calibrated measurements of scanned tissues with an image resolution in the order of less than one millimetre. Thus, pre-operative DVT of the larynx and on-site volume rendering, including 3D morphometry, enables the design of a unique optimally shaped silicone implant for medialization thyroplasty.

Method

Laryngeal DVT was performed having the patient in a seated position. The radiologic scanning of the larynx takes less than one minute (in high speed mode, approximately 15 seconds (see Figure 15.1)). The laryngeal cartilaginous framework configuration was directly imaged on a computer screen and is measured off-line through comparison with ultrasound images. The ideal shape of the implant was then drawn by superimposing onto a CT image, allowing a precise measurement of depth, length, and height of the implant. Thus, an individual-

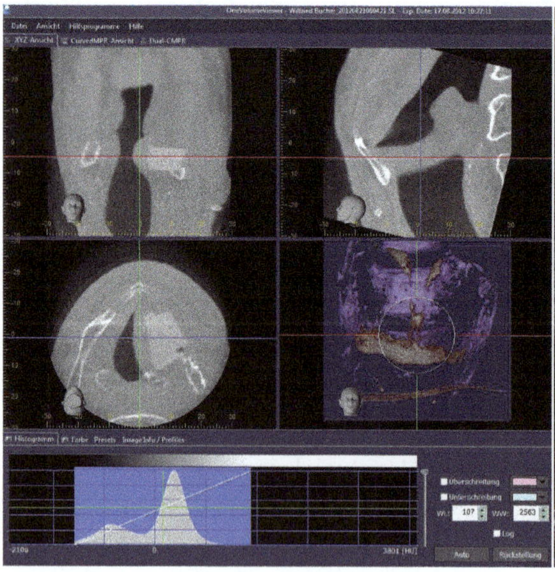

Figure 15.1: Precise measurement of cartilage size is possible with DVT scanning.

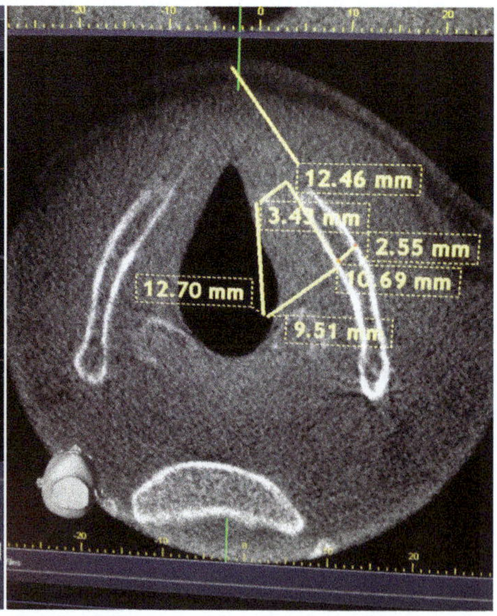

Figure 15.2: Pre-operative ideal implant size and shape are drawn onto the image.

ized, pre-operative, DVT-based morphometric ideal implant shape was calculated (Figure 15.2).

Results

Marked variations of thyroid cartilage angles and shapes were seen after DVT scanning. Knowledge of 'ideal' implant shapes, based on DVT imaging, was very helpful for intra-operative carving and positioning of the silicone implant. Results were verified by post-operative DVT and post-operative voice assessment, proving successful medialization. Swallowing during DVT image acquisition resulted in blurring of scans. In extreme cases, morphometry is then impossible. Thus, patients have to be instructed to avoid swallowing for the 15 to 50 seconds of scanning.

Discussion

Individualized implant design before medialization thyroplasty facilitated dimensions for the perfect shaping of an intra-operative carved silicone block. The most valuable information was the depth of the posterior part of the implant, which is crucial for medializing the vocal process. In cases of recurrent laryngeal nerve paralysis, medialization of the vocal process was the most important feature when 'constructing' the ideally shaped implant. It has been shown in another study that prefabricated ready-to-use implants did not always enable medialization of the vocal process (Figure 15.3).

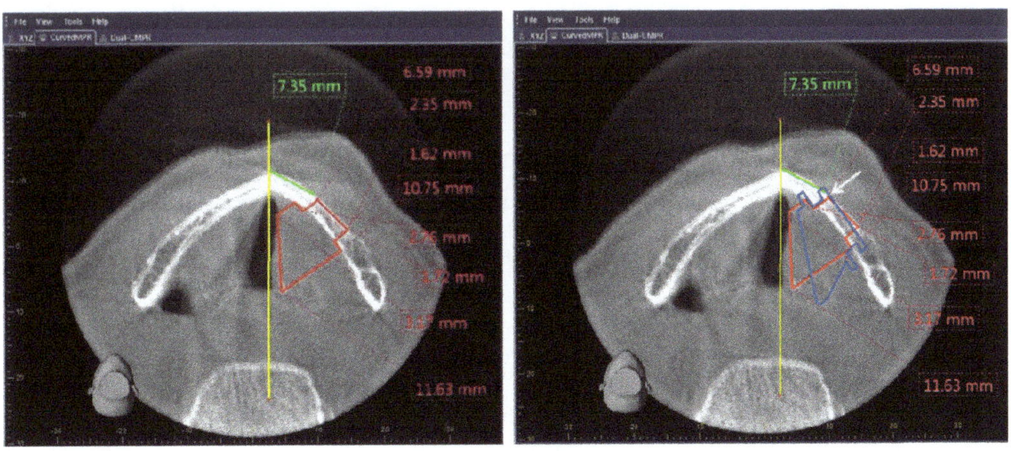

Figure 15.3: A screenshot is taken to the OR. Note that, with DVT, exact millimetre sizes of the larynx can be obtained. This would not be possible with MRI and CT scans. Good contrast between cartilage and soft tissues (DVT is usually not indicated for soft tissue diagnostics).

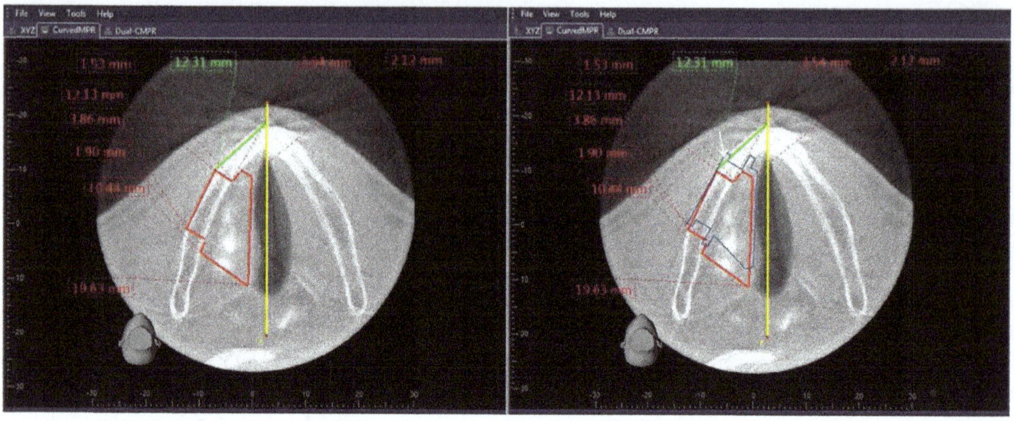

Figure 15.4: Post-operative implant morphometrical data can be pulled from the DVT scans via digital computer based measurements. Measurement and viewing from all sides, as well as 3D rotation features, facilitates visualization of implant location for the surgeon.

Furthermore, even in cases where pre-operative planning was not performed with DVT, it could be shown that post-operative assessment of implant position can be achieved with DVT (Figure 15.4).

Conclusion

In our patients marked individual variations of the three-dimensional laryngeal cartilage framing were seen. This justified the pre-operative individualized assessment and planning of implant shapes by examining the larynx with DVT.

String-pull technique for arytenoid adduction

Rationale

The purpose of this technique is to introduce a simplified surgical method for arytenoid adduction avoiding broad surgical exposure to access the muscular process of the arytenoid cartilage.

Methods

With an extra-intralaryngeally advanced 20G cannula, a non-absorbable 3-O mono-filament thread is placed and fixed next to the muscular process. The cannula and, finally, the 'string'-thread, lie in a direction such that its vector pull matches the pulling direction of the lateral cricoarytenoid muscle, resulting in a 'string-pull arytenoid adduction'. Figures 15.5 to 15.7 show how the cannula is placed transcutaneously in a superior, slightly lateral direction within the LCA muscle until it reaches the muscular process region. The needle keeps on advancing until it enters the pharyngeal lumen, so that the thread can be caught with a wire loop needle threader or, more simply, with a thread looped to catch the non-absorbable 3-O thread. Pulling out of the cannula with the looped wire/thread pulls the final 'string' thread with it. When the 'string' thread has several (8–12) knots at its other end, this thick knot-complex will anchor at the mus-

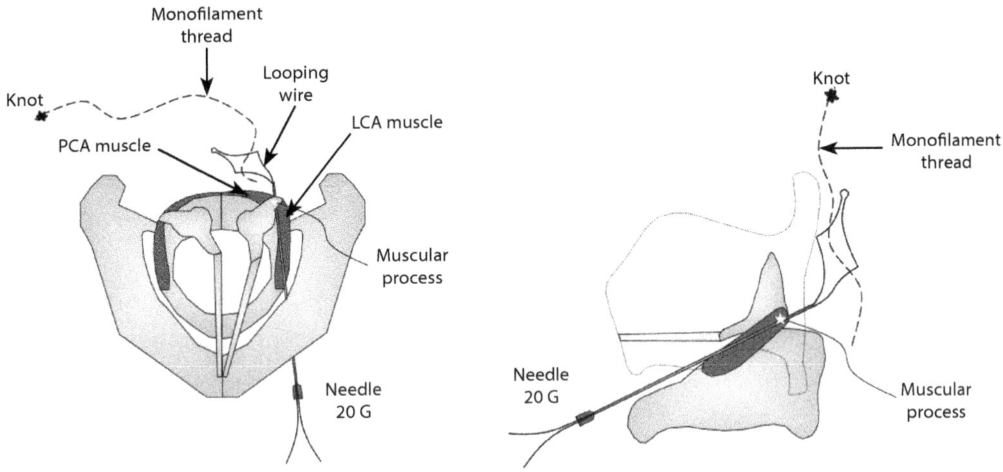

Figure 15.5: Percutaneously guided cannula and a wire loop needle threader catch a non-absorbable monofilament thread. Superior and lateral views.

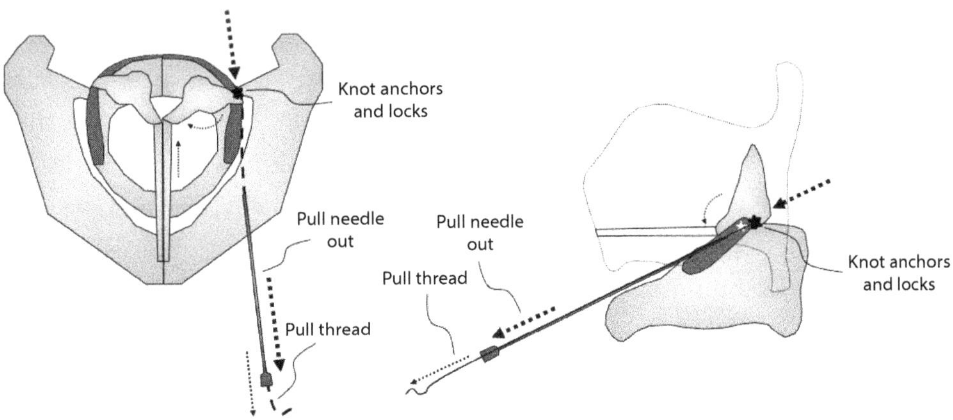

Figure 15.6: The thread is pulled through to anchor in the muscular process region. Superior and lateral views.

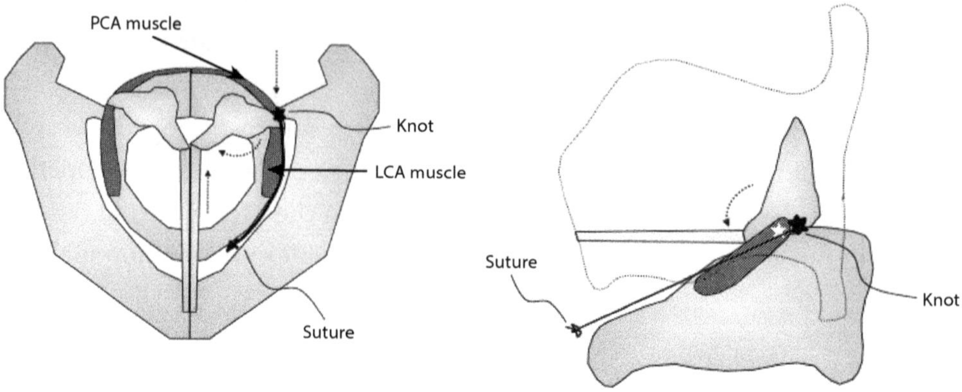

Figure 15.7: Continuous tension on the thread imitates the lateral cricoarytenoid muscle (LCA) action, resulting in a 'string-pull arytenoid adduction'. Superior and lateral views.

cular process and will not follow through the canal where the cannula passed. Thus, continuous pull on the 'string' thread will force the muscular process to follow, resulting in an arytenoid adduction while resembling the action of the LCA muscle.

Discussion

After successfully adopting the principle using excised human larynges, we were able to prove in three cases (with patients consenting to undergo the procedure under general anaesthesia) that this technique achieved arytenoid rotation. Here, string-pull arytenoid adduction resulted in a significant post-operative arytenoid rotation. The rotational effect following string-pull arytenoid adduction is similar to conventional arytenoid adduction. In our patients, the string-pull arytenoid adduction was made in combination with medialization thyroplasty with individually carved implants. Theoretically, it should be possible to perform such an operation in the office. A percutaneous approach can be used with a 20 G cannula, using simultaneous transnasal flexible endoscopy with instruments to help feed the string-thread into the catching loop visible at the posterior part of the arytenoid hump.

Conclusion

String-pull arytenoid adduction has the advantage that it is performed from an external approach and avoids making a cartilage window or excising parts of the cartilage. It also avoids an open-larynx access to reach the muscular process. Further studies should assess the clinical value of this technique.

Pin-up glottoplasty

Rationale

Thyroplasty is the gold standard procedure for permanently medializing a unilaterally paralysed vocal fold. However, thyroplasty surgery necessitates open neck surgery with a significant exposure and windowing of the thyroid ala. The idea of pin-up glottoplasty is to minimize surgical exposure of the larynx just to the anterior aspect and avoid drilling a bigger window. In this procedure a sagitally placed wire passes from anterior to posterior 'holding' the immobile vocal fold permanently in a median position. The same pin-up technique can be used in cases of bilateral vocal fold paralysis, where lateralization of the vocal fold would be the surgical target and the posterior wire fixation is in a lateral position. This has been investigated in cadaveric excised human larynges.

Methods

Pin-up glottoplasty uses a stiff, straight wire (e.g. titanium) that is advanced through an anterior thyroid ala hole after making a minimal skin incision and drill-hole in the anterior thyroid ala with a small burr (maximum 1 mm). The drill-hole position is similar (albeit more lateral) to Steven Gray's minithyrotomy approach. The wire is passed through the hole from anterior to posterior, strictly inside the vocal fold (but not in Reinke's space), preferably alongside the vocal ligament/vocalis muscle in a paramedial and saggital direction. Making sure that the vocal fold is kept in a median (adducted) position, the wire is finally advanced more posteriorly until it passes the vocal process and ends inside the posterior cricoid cartilage (Figure 15.8). More specifically, the wire punches into the cricoid cartilage, and

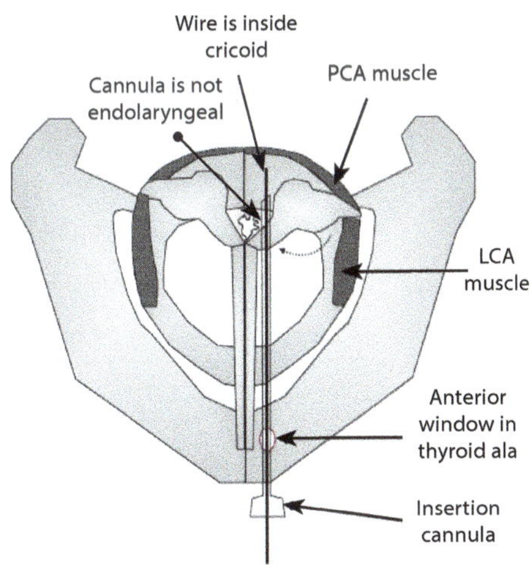

Figure 15.8: A cannula is advanced saggitally, totally intrachordally and alongside an immobile vocal fold, from anterior to posterior, until it reaches the cricoid cartilage.

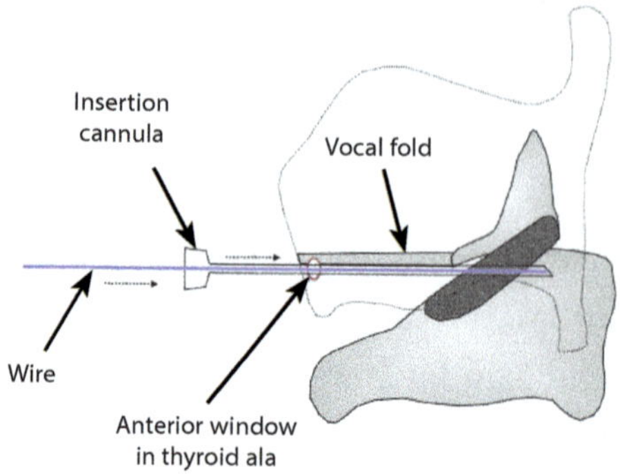

Figure 15.9: Once the wire is fixed inside the cricoid, it resembles a 'pinning-up' of the wire, resulting in a stabilized wire fixation and thus static position of the pinned up vocal fold.

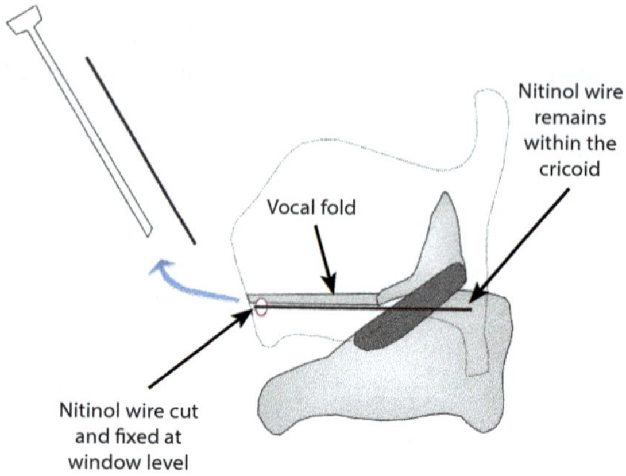

Figure 15.10: When the wire is pinned up paramedian, the vocal fold is forced to stay medial and the effect is a medialization glottoplasty.

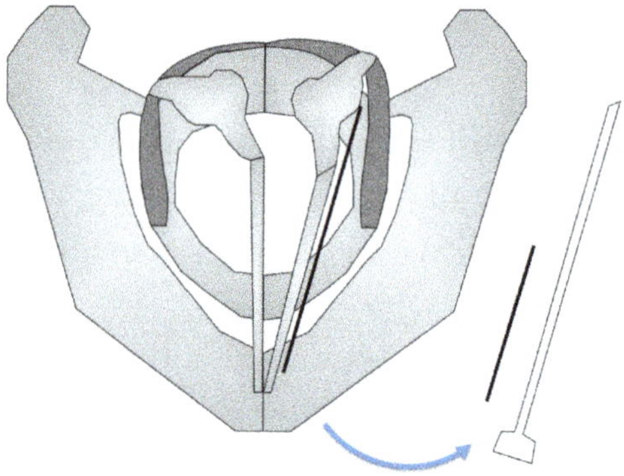

Figure 15.11: However, when the wire is pinned up laterally, it would keep the vocal fold abducted, resembling a lateralization glottoplasty.

stops as soon as it is inside the cricoid. After posterior positioning is completed, the wire is fixed anteriorly, e.g. with a screw or mini-plate. Due to the intracordal stiffness of the wire, the vocal fold will remain in a straight, rigid and stable position (Figure 15.9).

During the advancement of the wire through the vocal fold, the procedure will need endolaryngeal visual control for making sure that the wire is strictly staying inside the vocal fold, maintaining a median position and avoiding endoluminal perforation of the wire, especially in the posterior part between vocal process and cricoid cartilage. Because the posterior insertion point of the wire is of crucial importance for voice outcome, placement of the wire at the final 'pin-up' position needs fine adjustment and visual control. This is not only for the medial-to-lateral position, but also for the correct inferior-to-superior level. Therefore, observing the advancement of the wire during microlaryngoscopy with jet ventilation would be appropriate.

Pre-operative digital volume tomography (DVT) of the larynx may facilitate the operation by providing morphometrical data on thyroid and cricoid cartilage shapes and sizes, and thickness of the posterior cartilage plate. This also allows for exact determination of the length of the wire.

Discussion

The paramedian position and stiffness of the intraligament wire will enable a favourable phonatory function. The stability of the wire position is ensured by the well-chosen fixation points anteriorly and posteriorly (Figures 15.10 and 15.11).

To avoid post-operative infections through any endoluminal passage of the wire, it is of importance to make sure that the entire wire is covered by tissue and thus stays within the vocal fold and posterior laryngeal mucosa during the advancement procedure. While advancing the wire through the membranous part of the vocal fold, laryngoscopic visualization of subtle wiggling movements of the wire tip facilitate observation of strict intracordal wire advancement.

Preferably, the tip of the wire should be sharp and stiff enough to allow penetration into the cricoid cartilage; a thickened tip part can facilitate long term anchoring inside of the cricoid cartilage. Titanium would be a good candidate for such an implant due to its biological tolerability and anti-magnetic properties for MRI tomography.

When implants are designed, there should always be an easy way to remove them without damaging the tissues. Thus, instead of hooking the wire inside of the cricoid (which would indeed give a better fixation and keep the implant from migration), the wire should be kept straight at the posterior part for potential explant cases.

This method of pin-up glottoplasty could also allow for a lateralization procedure in cases of bilateral vocal fold paralysis, but in this case the posterior fixation point would be chosen at a very lateral cricoid point.

Conclusion

With an intracordal stiff wire pinned up at a paramedian position in the cricoid cartilage, a straight and stable position of the entire vocal fold is ensured. Thus, it is conceivable that medialization glottoplasty (or lateralization glottoplasty, if wanted) may be performed with such a less invasive approach. More studies in excised larynges and future clinical investigations are needed to prove if this approach can be an alternative to state-of-art medialization thyroplasty techniques, or in cases of bilateral paralysis, for vocal fold lateralization.

Anti-stridor Nitinol needle

Rationale

The purpose of this technique is to introduce an instrument for possible future office-based vocal fold lateralization in patients with bilateral vocal fold immobility and stridor. Through a percutaneous lateral cricothytroid membrane approach, a cannula containing a Nitinol® wire with memory effect for an anterior hook shape is advanced into the supraglottal space. When the Nitinol wire is pushed out of the cannula, its tip bends around the vocal fold: the wire 'hooks' on the vocal fold, so that a lateral pull at the outer wire leads to a lateralization of the immobile vocal fold. A prototype was manufactured and the applicability of the technique was proven in excised human larynges.

Methods

From an external approach, a curved Nitinol wire with memory effect, resting inside the lumen of a cannula, is forwarded through a percutaneous approach externally through the lateral cricothyroid membrane, passing through the paraglottal tissue space and intruding into the lumen of Morgagni's ventricle, finally ending in the supraglottic lumen. Advancement of the wire out of the cannula tip leads to curving of the wire around the vocal fold due to the memory effect of Nitinol. The size of the Nitinol wire bend can be determined by the manufacturer and is therefore predictable. In an office setting, the wire placement may be visualized through flexible laryngoscopy, and fine adjustments for hooking onto the vocal fold are enabled without the need for microlaryngoscopy in general anaesthesia. Once the hook is placed around the vocal fold, soft wire pull lateralizes the vocal fold and widens the glottis, as can be visualized and controlled by laryngoscopy. Fixation of the outer Nitinol wire can be accomplished by several means, e.g. by fixing the wire with a mini-plate and a conical screw nut (Figure 15.12).

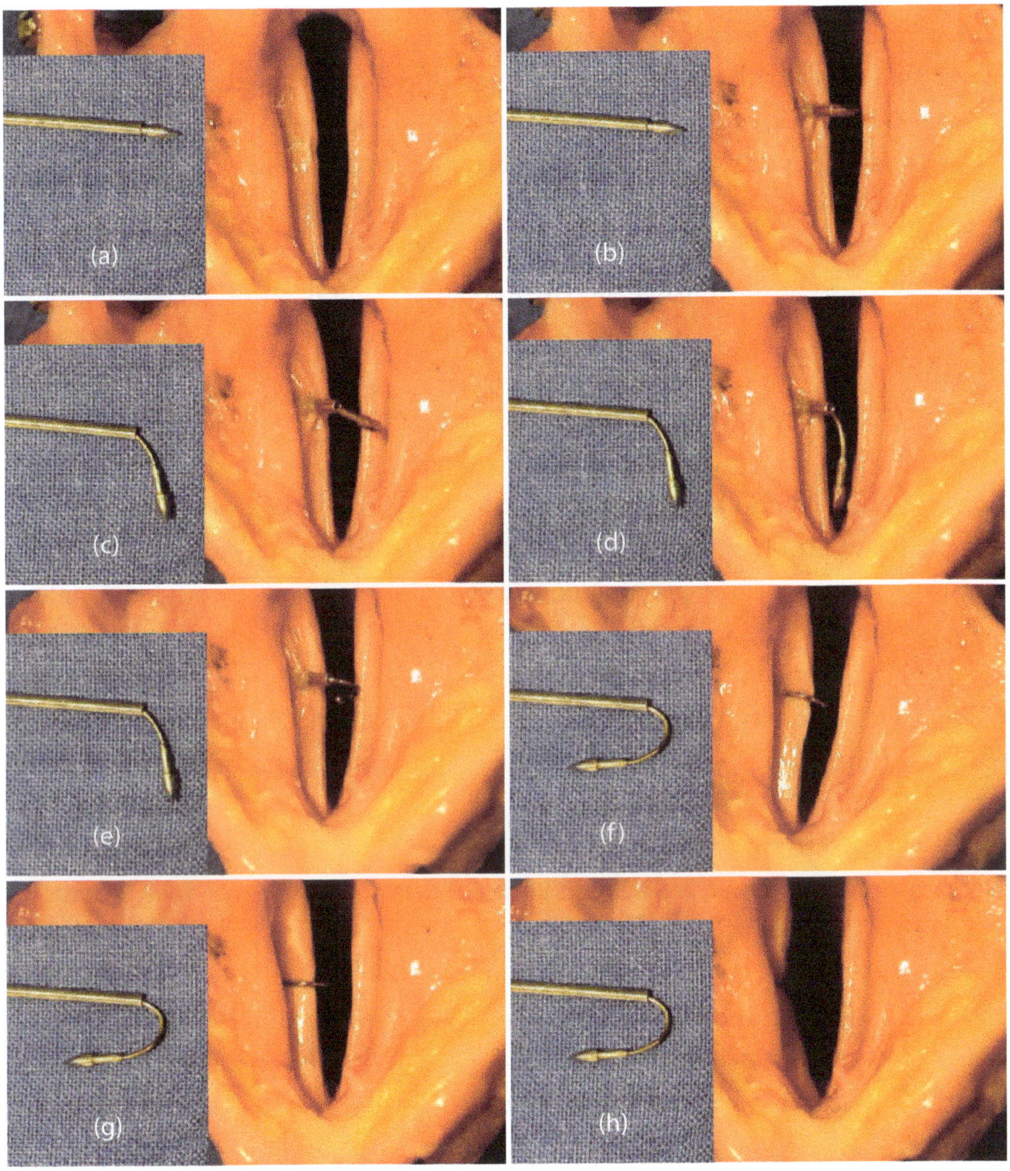

Figure 15.12: Lateralization via external approach. A cannula containing a Nitinol wire with a sharp tip is advanced through the lateral aspect of the cricothyroid membrane (a). As soon as the needle tip is visualized endolaryngeally (b), the Nitinol wire is pushed into the supraglottal space, resulting in curving of the wire (c, d). After rotating the wire tip downwards (e), the wire is pushed further and curves approx. 180° (f, g). Now retraction of wire pulls the vocal fold laterally and inferiorly, resulting in opening of the glottis (h).

Results

We proved the applicability of the technique in excised larynx experiments. External pull on the crook-shaped wire resulted in vocal fold lateralization and glottic widening. It was easier to set the cannula through the lateral cricothyroid space than transcartilaginous through the thyroid cartilage. The upright angulation of the cannula needs to be quite steep and at least 45° from the horizontal plane to safely reach the Morgagni's ventricle. The procedure can be performed within one minute when the wire tip is visualized via laryngoscopy. After lateralization, the triangular shape of the glottis now resembles the glottal area shape that would also result if using the Lichtenberger lateralization technique.

Discussion

The idea of an 'anti-stridor' needle is meant as a possible emergency tool for an ENT office. In cases of bilateral vocal fold immobility when the supralarynx is not swollen, the endolarynx can be visualized via rigid or flexible laryngoscopy. Given that the neck of the patient is not too thick, it should be possible to place and advance the device percutaneously in an angled way through the lateral cricothyroid space.

Once the glottal area is enlarged, the wire can be fixed externally, keeping the glottis open. The physician now has time to make a decision how to proceed, e.g. performing a non-emergency tracheotomy or choosing other measures for a safe airway.

Further investigations, e.g. finding the ideal wire thickness and bend that works for most patients, are needed to make this a ready-to-use instrument.

Conclusion

This technique has the potential for application as an office-based lateralization procedure in awake patients, avoiding emergency tracheotomy, intubation, or other measures. However, the device is not a long-term implant, such that the main advantage is to get quick airway control and gain time for decision-making. Further studies should assess the clinical value of this technique.

Acknowledgements

It is widely acknowledged that 'ideas' mostly reflect a collective wisdom and sometimes one only needs a tiny spark to find a technique that can be applied in our phonosurgical field. In some cases, we only have to look for techniques that other colleagues use in their professions. The collaboration and support of many colleagues for the abovementioned applications is very much acknowledged and appreciated. Special thanks go to Susanne Fleischer, Reinhard Friedrich, Michael Kammal, Aiham Mousli, Frank Müller, Almut Niessen, Stefan Noster, Christina Pflug, and Klaus Püschel. The author thanks H. Grosse Company for designing and manufacturing the Nitinol needle.

Further reading

Friedrich G, Remacle M, Birchall M, et al. 2007. Defining phonosurgery: a proposal for classification and nomenclature by the Phonosurgery Committee of the European Laryngological Society (ELS). *Eur Arch Otorhinolaryngol* **264**(10):1191–1200.

Frizzarini R, Gebrim EM, Imamura R, et al. 2011. Individually customized implants for laryngoplasty – are they possible? *J Voice* **26**(5):619–22.

Hiramatsu H, Tokashiki R, Suzuki M. 2008. Usefulness of three-dimensional computed tomography of the larynx for evaluation of unilateral vocal fold paralysis before and after treatment: technique and clinical applications. *Eur Arch Otorhinolaryngol* **265**:725–30.

Von Bruns V. 1862. *Die erste Ausrottung eines Polypen in der Kehlkopfshöhle durch Zerschneiden ohne blutige Eröffnung der Luftwege nebst einer kurzen Anleitung zur Laryngoskopie.* Tübingen: Verlag der H. Laupp'schen Buhhandlung, Laupp & Siebeck.

Index

www.ingramcontent.com/pod-product-compliance
Ingram Content Group UK Ltd.
Pitfield, Milton Keynes, MK11 3LW, UK
UKHW052002041026
15590UKWH00008B/2102

9 781909 082076